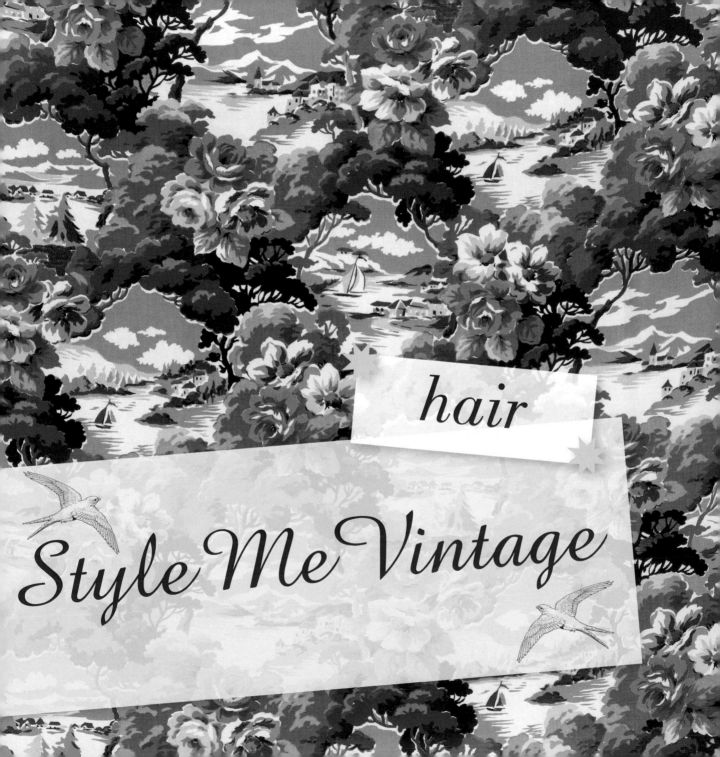

hair

Style Me Vintage

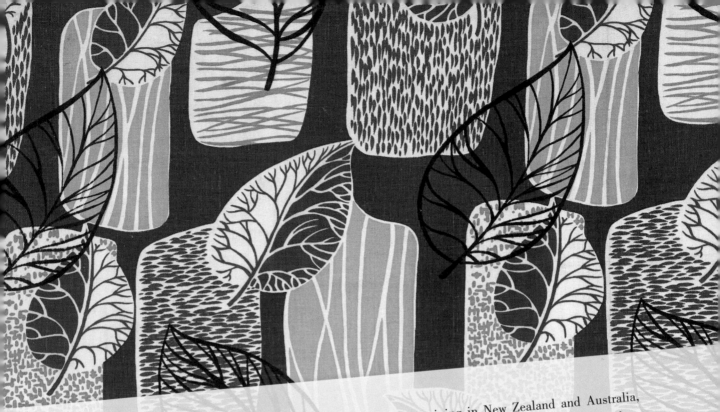

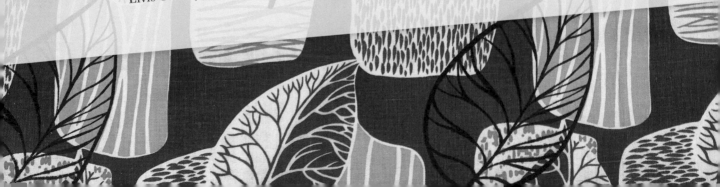

Belinda Hay is the founder of The Painted Lady, a unique boutique hair salon which specialises in vintage and contemporary colour, cuts and 'up do's' for ladies and gents.

With over 12 years international expertise, Belinda's passion for all things vintage started at the tender age of five with an infatuation with Elvis Presley and 1950's fashion. After many years training in New Zealand and Australia, she worked for some of London's top hair salons before opening her own charismatic salon based in London's Shoreditch. She now creates signature cuts and styles beautifully tailored to clients seeking an 'of the moment' retro look.

www.paintedladylondon.com

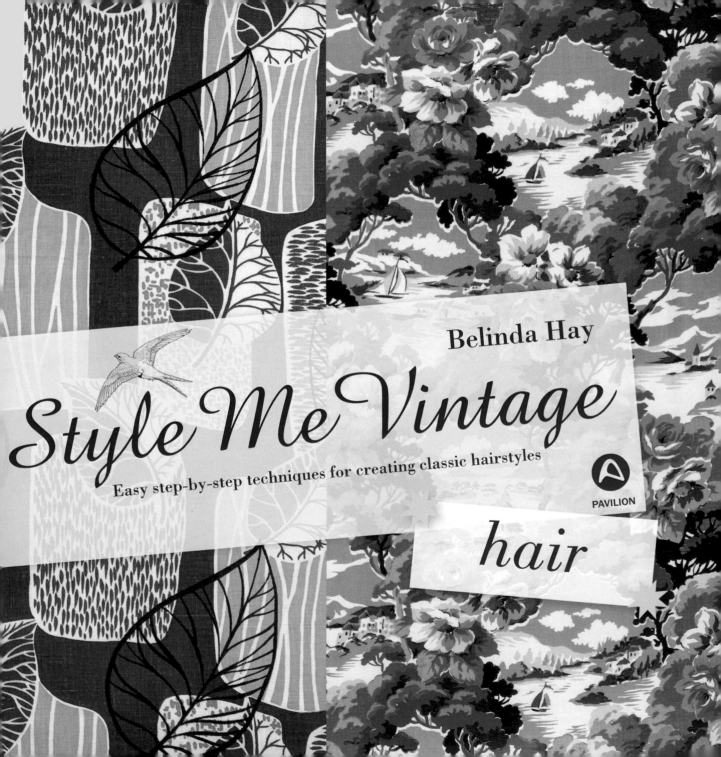

Belinda Hay

Style Me Vintage

Easy step-by-step techniques for creating classic hairstyles

PAVILION

hair

First published in the United Kingdom in 2010 by
PAVILION BOOKS
10 Southcombe Street, London W14 0RA

An imprint of Anova Books Company Ltd

Text © Belinda Hay, 2010
Design and layout © Anova Books, 2010
Photography © Anova Books, 2010,
except those images listed in Picture Credits page 111

Commissioning Editor: Emily Preece-Morrison
Designer: Georgina Hewitt
Photographer: Caroline Molloy
Hair stylist: Belinda Hay
Clothing stylist: Susan Downing
Makeup: Luisa Savoia using MAC
Models: Siren Stiletto, Jaime McLennan, Jessica de Lotz, Bao Reinke,
Jo Heygate and Rebecca Johnson
Production: Oliver Jeffreys

ISBN: 978-1-86205-902-3

A CIP catalogue record for this book is available from the British Library.

10 9 8 7 6 5 4

Colour reproduction by Rival Colour Ltd., UK
Printed and bound by Canale, Italy

www.anovabooks.com

Contents

Introduction

Have you ever wanted to primp and coiffure your hair to perfection? Or been inspired by the golden ages of fashion and silver screen goddesses? Hairstyles throughout the decades have been the foundation of many a vintage look, but the techniques used to create them, once taken for granted, are now fading from modern girls' repertoires.

In this book you will find step-by-step techniques for achieving perfect pompadours, outrageous beehives and other essential styles to help transform yourself into a vintage vixen. I've included some of the most iconic hairstyles that made their mark over the decades to become the most inspiring and influential looks of the last century.

Remember though, be patient! Some of these styles take a bit of practise to master. Even the most skilled of hairstylists don't always get it right first time!

EXPERIMENT

Each technique given is just a guide. There are many different ways to personalise your vintage 'do'. Try rolling your barrel curls or pin curls in a different direction, for instance. You may find something that really works for you.

THE HAIRCUT

Your haircut is important. The cut that makes it easiest to create a vintage look is a simple one-length style, perhaps with a few soft layers through the bottom of your hair. That's not to say that more modern and heavily layered hairstyles cannot be transformed into an immaculately coiffed victory roll or a perfect peek-a-boo. It's just a little easier with a classic cut.

Some of the retro styles suit a fringe, others work better without. You have to decide what works best for you in terms of having a fringe cut or not.

Good luck and have fun!

Belinda

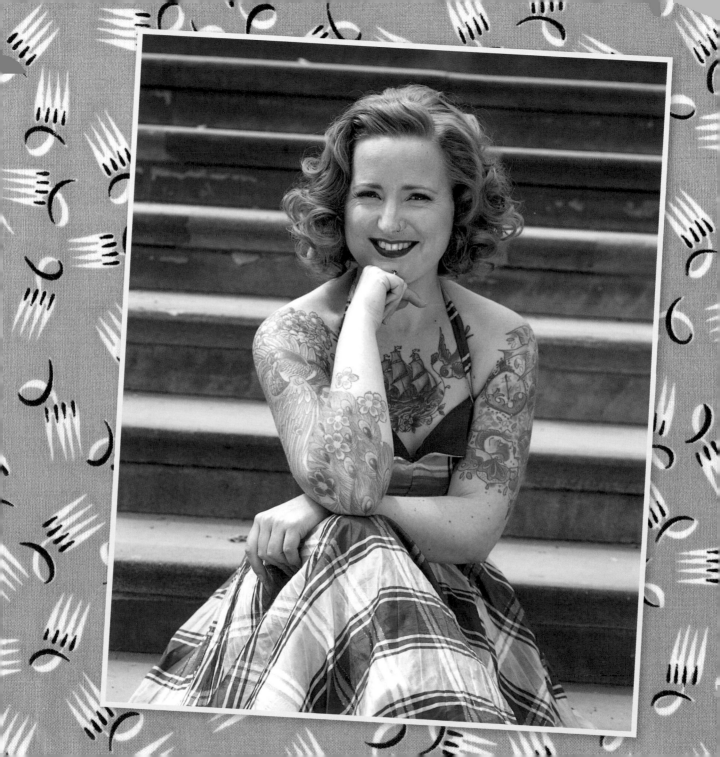

Essential Equipment

There are a number of 'essential' items you will need to help you create your vintage look, which I have listed over the following pages. You can mostly find these at hairdressing suppliers, department stores and chemists. However, you won't necessarily need all of these items at once. With time and experience you can usually modify techniques to suit your hairdressing style and the available equipment.

Sectioning clips, combs and brushes are definitely essential for creating most styles. To help you further, at the beginning of each style in this book, I have included a list of the equipment that you will need.

Decorative items are always lovely to add to your finished your style. Try fresh or silk flowers, a string of pearls or pretty hair clips, depending on what look you are after. Scarves and ribbons can also be used to give your style an extra special retro touch. See pages 100–107 for tips on styling retro scarves. Don't forget that hats were often an essential part of vintage outfits. Try adding a little pillbox hat to your bouffant to complete your look.

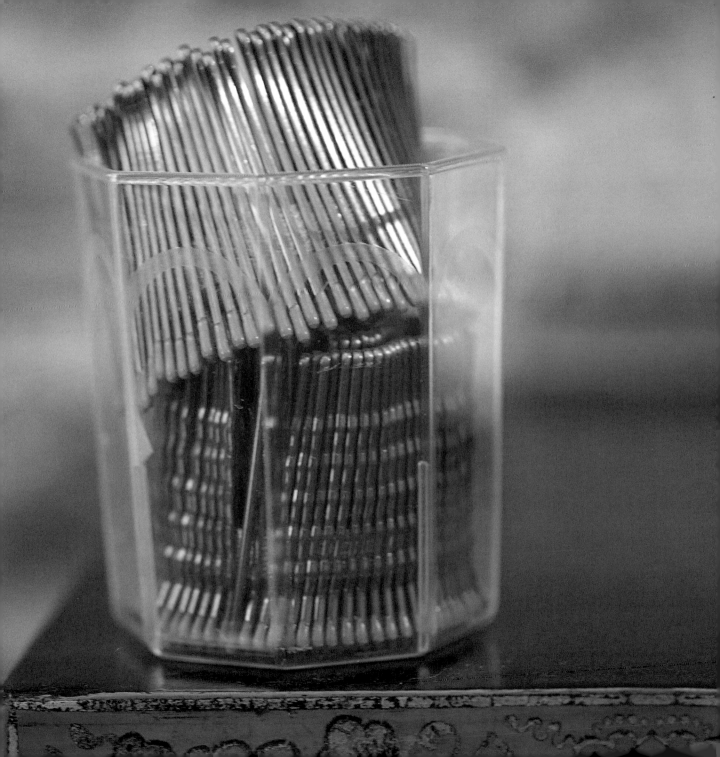

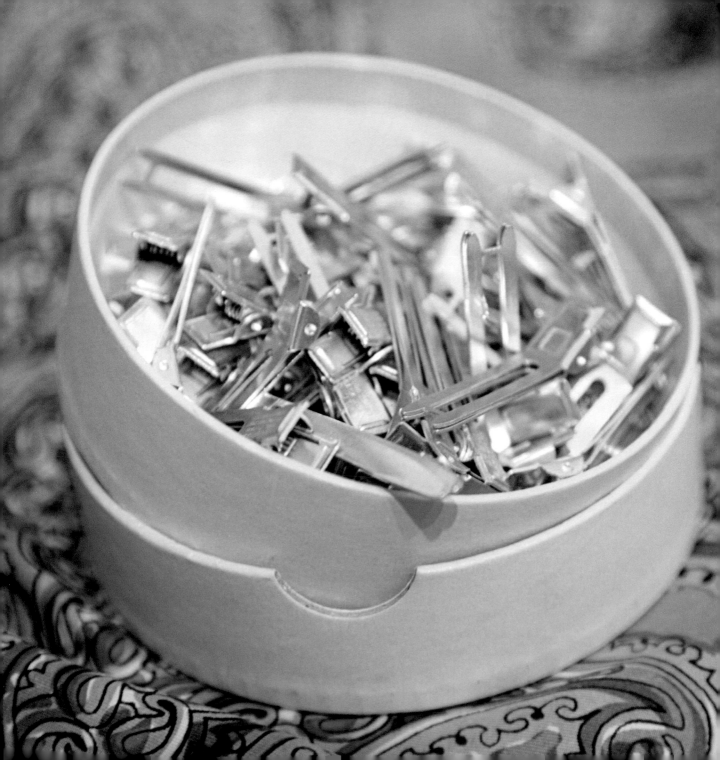

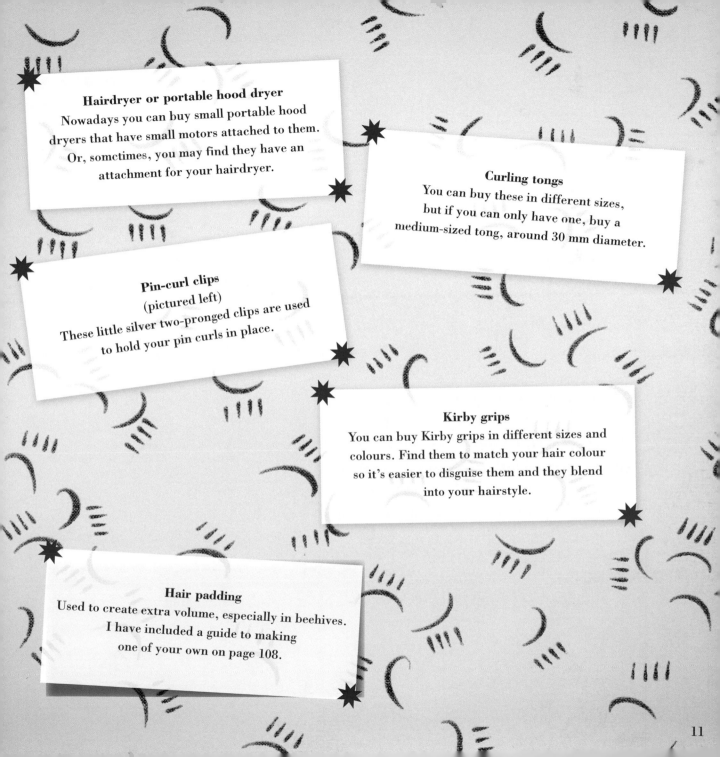

Hairdryer or portable hood dryer
Nowadays you can buy small portable hood dryers that have small motors attached to them. Or, somctimes, you may find they have an attachment for your hairdryer.

Curling tongs
You can buy these in different sizes, but if you can only have one, buy a medium-sized tong, around 30 mm diameter.

Pin-curl clips
(pictured left)
These little silver two-pronged clips are used to hold your pin curls in place.

Kirby grips
You can buy Kirby grips in different sizes and colours. Find them to match your hair colour so it's easier to disguise them and they blend into your hairstyle.

Hair padding
Used to create extra volume, especially in beehives. I have included a guide to making one of your own on page 108.

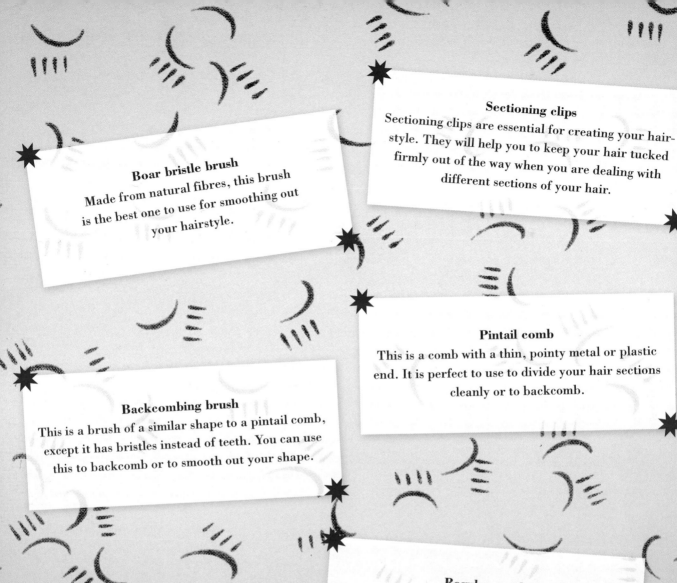

Boar bristle brush
Made from natural fibres, this brush is the best one to use for smoothing out your hairstyle.

Sectioning clips
Sectioning clips are essential for creating your hairstyle. They will help you to keep your hair tucked firmly out of the way when you are dealing with different sections of your hair.

Backcombing brush
This is a brush of a similar shape to a pintail comb, except it has bristles instead of teeth. You can use this to backcomb or to smooth out your shape.

Pintail comb
This is a comb with a thin, pointy metal or plastic end. It is perfect to use to divide your hair sections cleanly or to backcomb.

Regular comb
This is the best comb to gently comb out knots and tangles after you have shampooed and conditioned your hair.

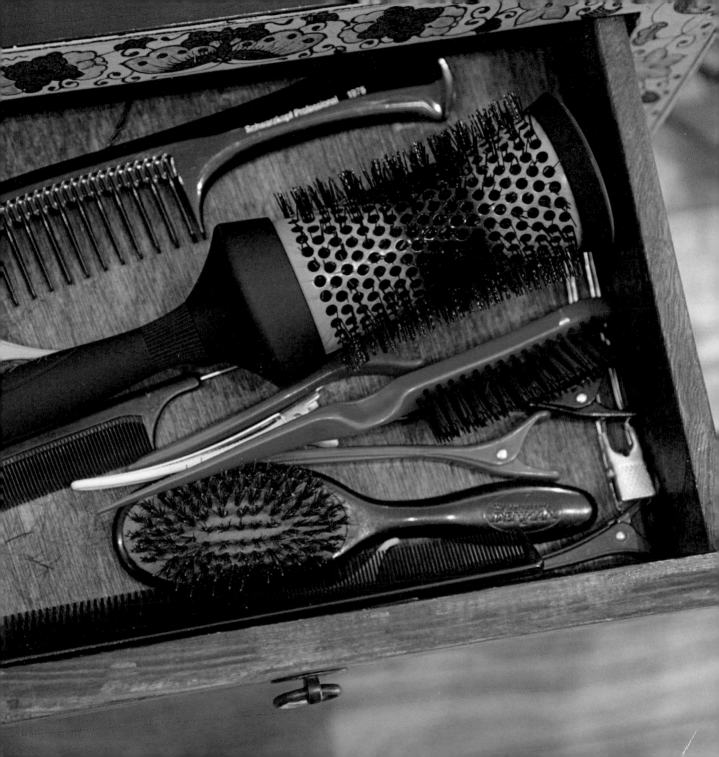

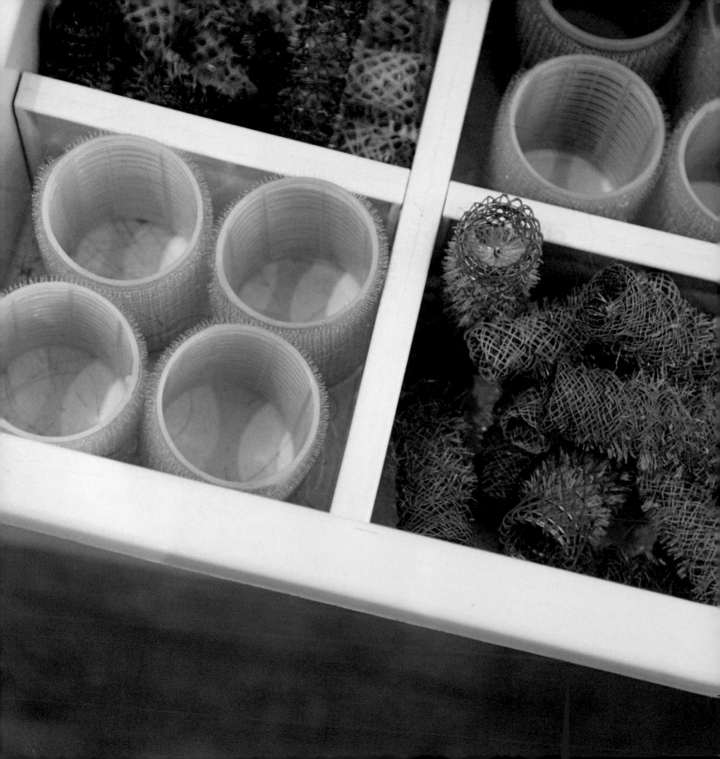

Rollers (various sizes)

You can use these to 'wet-set' your hair, or roll up sections as you are blow drying to create extra volume. Velcro rollers are the most readily available. You need to buy these in a size that will allow your hair to be wrapped around the roller two and a half to three times.

Heated rollers

These are usually sold in packs of set sizes in department stores and hairdressing suppliers.

Hairspray

You will need plenty of this. Hairspray is essential to keep your hairstyle rock solid. It will also help to give your style volume and support.

Synthetic hair pieces

You can find these, readymade, in different sizes and shapes. The most common is a doughnut shape. You can cut them down to the size you require.

Hairnet

Hairnets are great for protecting your hair overnight – to stop you getting 'bed head'; or you can use them to creating padding for your style.

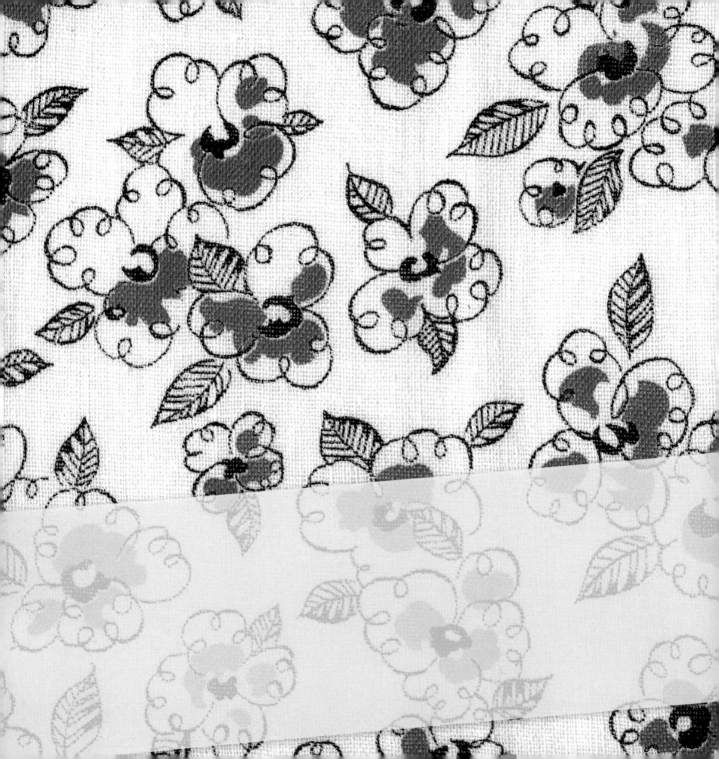

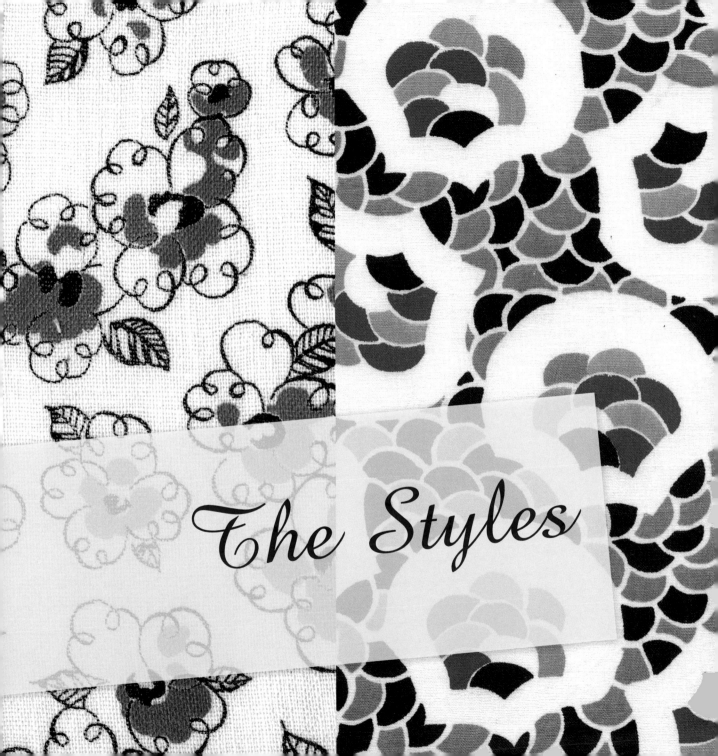

The Styles

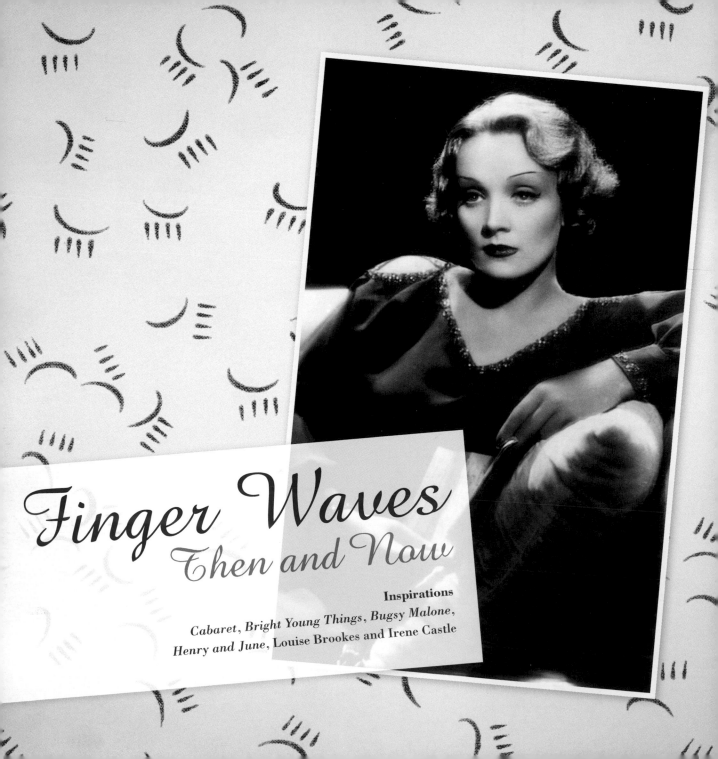

Finger Waves
Then and Now

Inspirations

Cabaret, Bright Young Things, Bugsy Malone,
Henry and June, Louise Brookes and Irene Castle

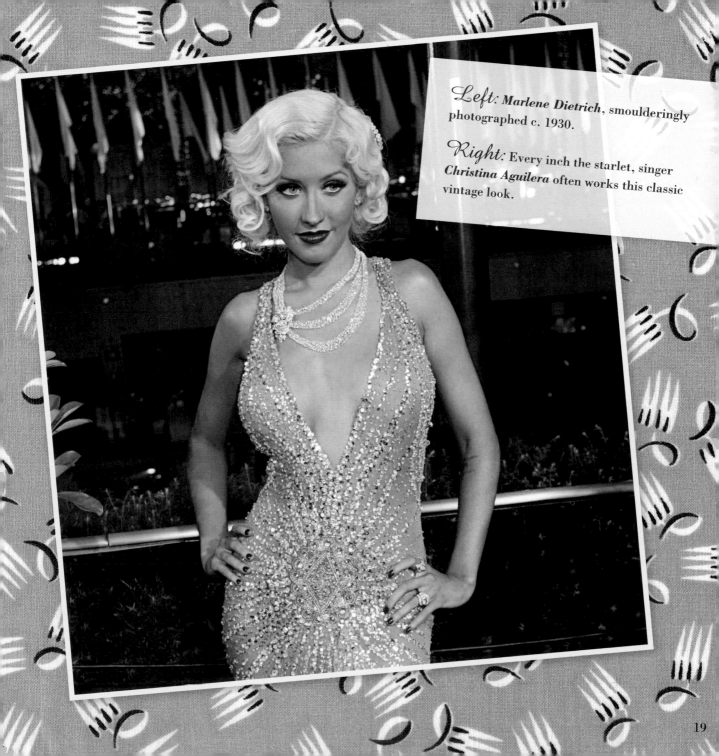

Left: **Marlene Dietrich**, smoulderingly photographed c. 1930.

Right: Every inch the starlet, singer **Christina Aguilera** often works this classic vintage look.

19

Finger Waves & Pin Curls

During the flapper era, fashions were boyish. Women's figures were hidden beneath straight-cut dresses, hemlines became shorter and so did hair lengths. Cropped bobs became very popular in the 1920s, but were first seen in Hollywood on the American actress Irene Castle, who had worn her hair in this way as early as 1914. Finger waves were often used to soften the masculine edge of a bob.

The difference between a finger wave and a Marcel wave is that finger waves, also known as water waves, are created on wet hair, whereas a Marcel wave is created by using heat on dry hair. Finger waves were often seen alongside pin curls, which were almost always used to style and finish the ends of the hair. In old-fashioned hairdressing, the general rule was to have 3 waves and 2 rows of pin curls.

You will need
Styling products, such as gel, mousse or setting lotion
Barbering comb
Pin-curl clips
Water spray bottle
A portable dryer
(you can buy these from hairdressing suppliers and some department stores)
Boar bristle brush

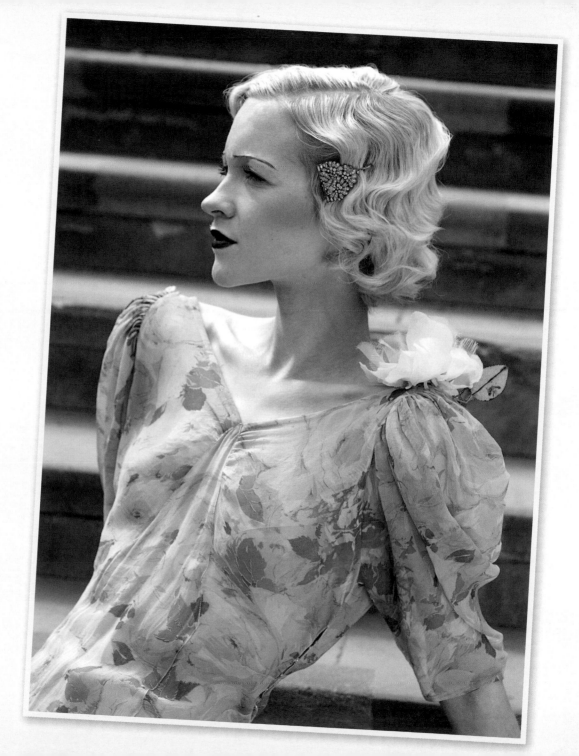

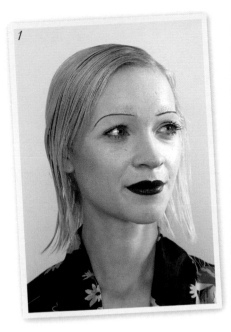

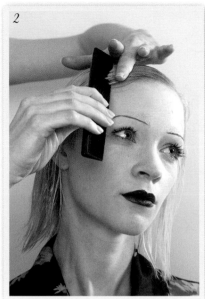

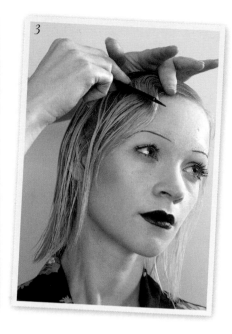

Finger waves are usually styled on hair that is shoulder length or shorter. You may find it easier to have a friend help you to create this style.

Step 1
Shampoo and towel dry your hair.

Step 2
Apply a generous amount of setting lotion, mousse or gel. Your hair needs to remain completely saturated throughout the styling process for the fingerwaves to be successful.

Step 3
Part your hair on your preferred side and comb it through, distributing the hair evenly and in a natural fall around your head (Fig.1). It is important for the hair to be distributed evenly so that there is enough hair for each row of finger waves.

Step 4
Comb your hair back away from your hair line (Fig. 2). You are going to create a 'c' shape. Place your middle finger flat along your scalp where you wish to make your first wave. Apply pressure with your middle finger so you don't disturb the hair you have already combed back to start your 'c' and comb the hair smoothly in a downwards motion.

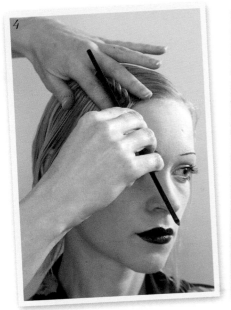
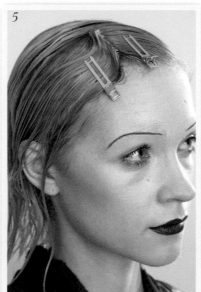
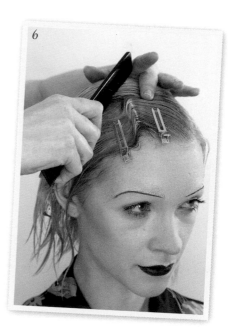

Step 5

Once the hair is combed through smoothly, keeping your middle finger in place, comb the hair forwards (Fig.3). At this stage your comb should be in an upright position.

Step 6

Once you have begun to comb the hair forward in a 'c' shape, you need to flatten the comb to your scalp and push up towards your middle finger. Once you reach the middle finger with your comb, lift the comb back to an upright position (Fig. 4). This will create the crest of the wave. Keeping your middle finger fixed on your scalp, place your index finger on the other side of the upright comb. Now you have your middle and index fingers both applying pressure on the scalp – one finger on either side of the comb.

Step 7

With your pin-curl clips, pin either side of the crest lifting your fingers up slightly so the grips can slide into place (Fig.5).

Step 8

It is very important to make sure your hair has been combed in a natural fall so you don't have gaps in your crests and waves. Make a second crest and wave behind the first one using the same techniques from steps 4 to 7. You need to place your middle finger in line with the first placing so that you can make the crests join together in the second wave (Fig.6).

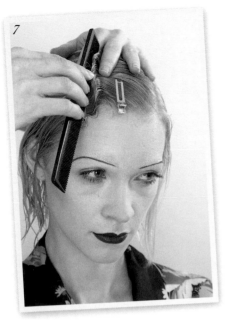

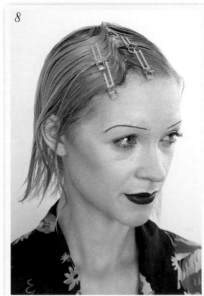

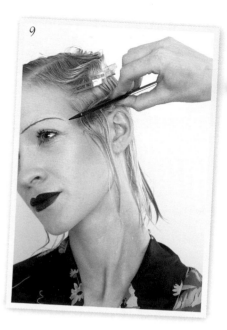

Step 9
Form the second crest as before in line with the first, and place clips either side (Figs.7 and 8).

Step 10
Continue this all the way around the head through the crown until you reach the other hairline.

Step 11
Start the second row of waves from the opposite hairline using the same technique (steps 4 to 10), although this time you will be creating a 'backwards c' (Fig. 9). Continue this all the way around the head again to the opposite hairline. You need to continue to make runs of curls until you get to the occipital bone, where your head dips in to the nape of your neck.

Pin curls
(steps 12 to 15)
You can use this technique with finger waves or on its own, pin-curling your entire head of hair. Pin curls are a fundamental part of vintage hairstyling and the essence of this technique is adapted and used in different forms throughout this book.

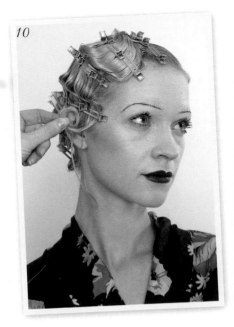
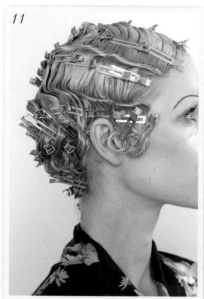
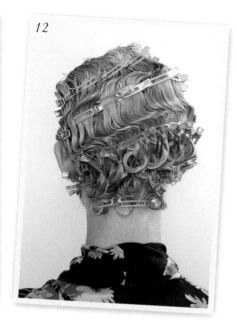

Step 12

Now you have some lengths of hair that are loose at the end of your fingerwaves. Take up a row of hair at the bottom of the fingerwaves about 2 cm wide. You are going to split this into sections about 2 cm thick. This can be done as you go along, creating a small, square base for your pin curl to sit on.

Step 13

Each row of pin curls should be curled in the same direction. Let's call them 'b'-shaped and 'd'-shaped.

Look at the direction of your last wave – 'c' or 'backwards c'. This will determine which way your pin curl will be placed as you need to continue creating a flowing waveform.

If your last fingerwave was a 'c' shape, your next pin curl will be a 'd' shape. Likewise, a 'backwards c' should follow with a 'b' shape pin curl.

You need to take the hair from your small square section and, holding the very tips of your hair between your forefinger and thumb, and alternating your left and right hand, begin to roll up the curl towards the base of the section (Fig. 10). Always hold the ends of your hair in the curl with thumb and forefinger. You will see how the pin curl will look like a 'b' or 'd' shape.

Step 14

Once you have rolled up your pin curl , use a pin-curl clip to secure the curl in place. The clip needs to be placed into the curl at and through the base, so it is holding the curl firmly (Fig. 11).

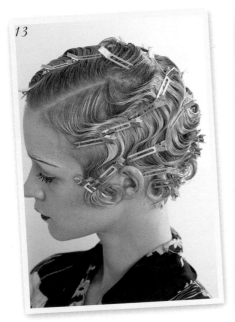

13

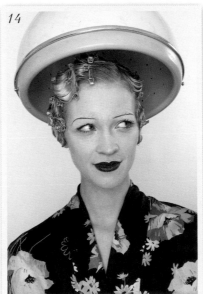

14

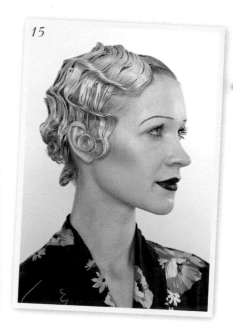

15

Step 15

Finish the row of pin curls and start the next row, but this time you need to curl your pin curls in the opposite direction to the last row. This will continue the wave through to the end (Figs. 12 and 13).

Step 16

Dry your hair (Fig. 14).

You can let your hair dry naturally, although this could take some time depending on the thickness of your hair – up to 12 hours. Alternatively, you can sit under a portable soft dryer. You can find these at department stores and hairdressing suppliers. Under a dryer the process could take up to 45 minutes, depending on your hair thickness.

*It is very important to make sure your finger waves are bone dry. If there is a hint of moisture in your hair when you come to brush them out, you will lose the wave.

Step 17

Once your hair is completely dry, remove all of the clips from your hair and start to brush out. You need to start from the bottom, using your fingers to push the waves back into place.

You could also leave your hair untouched if you would like a sleek, wet look (Fig. 15).

Step 18

Spray with hairspray to hold.

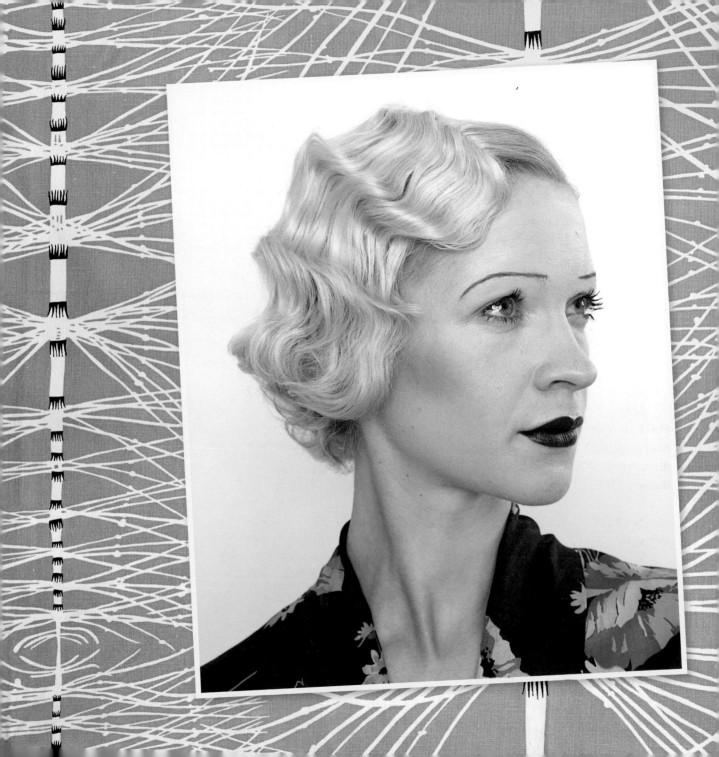

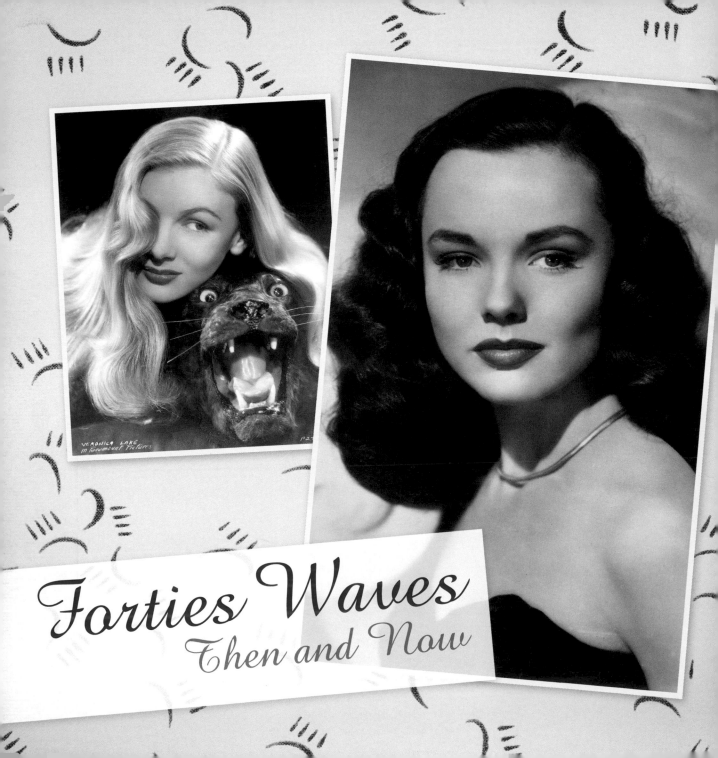

VERONICA LAKE
in Paramount Pictures

Forties Waves
Then and Now

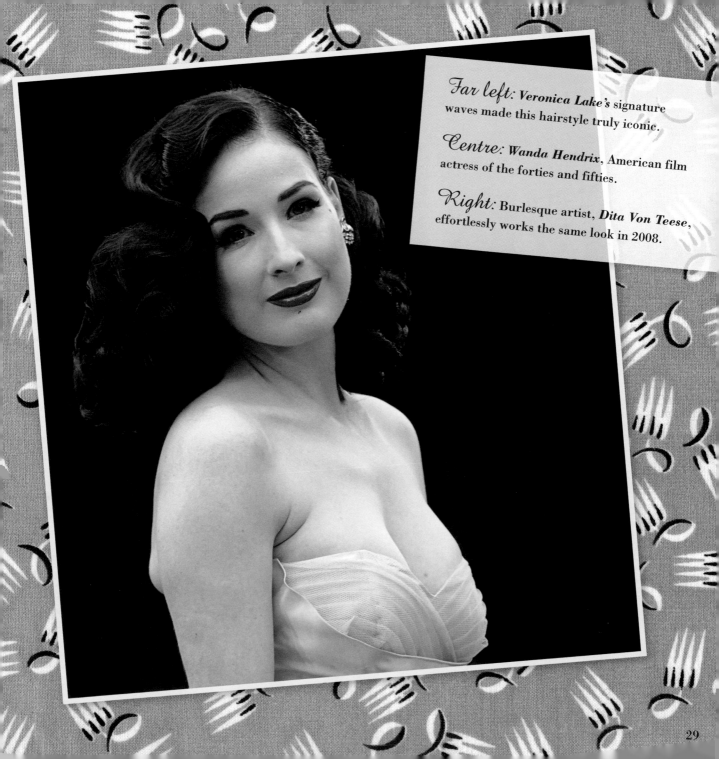

Far left: *Veronica Lake's* signature waves made this hairstyle truly iconic.

Centre: *Wanda Hendrix*, American film actress of the forties and fifties.

Right: Burlesque artist, *Dita Von Teese*, effortlessly works the same look in 2008.

29

The Peek-a-boo

Made famous by Veronica Lake, the peek-a-boo has been imitated and adapted by many of today's fashion icons. Considered one of the most seductive hairstyles, we see, again and again, modern sirens such as Dita Von Teese, Scarlett Johansson, Kim Basinger and Evan Rachel Wood pay tribute to this hairstyle's ability to transform them instantly into a silver-screen goddess…

A peek-a-boo is usually styled on hair that is shoulder length or longer.

You will need
Hairdryer
Round brushes
Curling tongs
Pin-curl clips
Hairspray
Comb
Soft bristle brush for smoothing

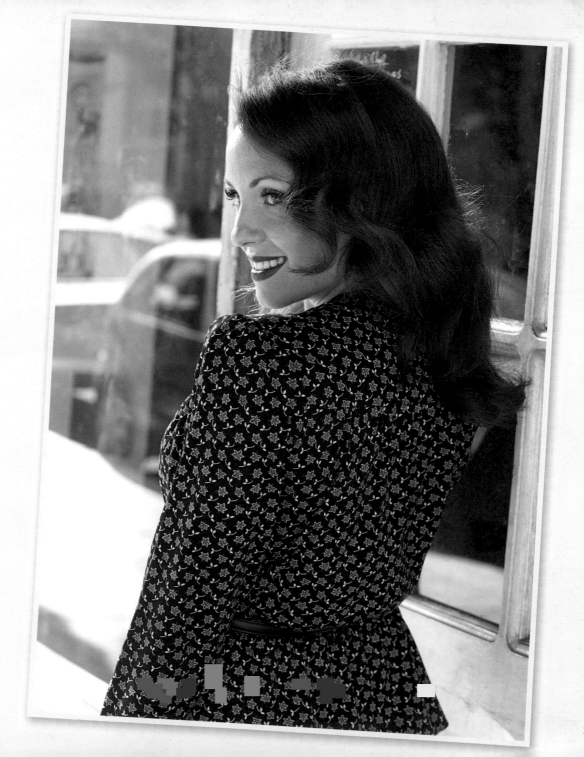

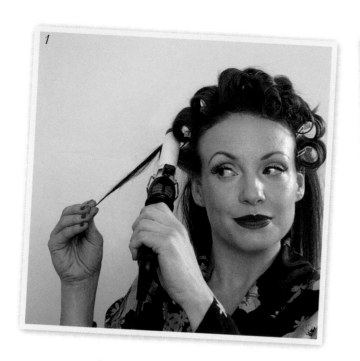

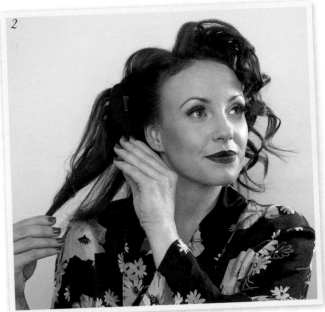

Step 1

Wash your hair and then blow dry your hair with volume. To increase volume, you can put rollers in your hair and blow dry, use heated rollers, or blow dry and pin your hair in rolls using pin-curl clips.

Step 2

Once your hair is blow-dried and curled up in the rollers or clips, spray with hairspray and leave for 10–15 minutes for it to cool down.

Step 3

Remove all of the rollers/clips and part your hair on the side. Choose the side that will give your hair the greatest volume for the wave at the top. Give it all another light hairspray.

Step 4

Brush out all of the curl with a soft padded brush (if you have hair that doesn't hold a curl well, it's best to miss out this step).

Step 5

Part your hair, taking your sections vertically and roughly 4 cm back from your front hairline.

Step 6

Take a small rectangular section on the heavy side of your parting, about 2 cm thick, and put your curling tongs in at the root (Fig. 1).

*Be careful not to burn yourself. Try resting a comb between the hot tongs and your scalp, so the tongs don't come into contact with your scalp.

Holding the mid-lengths of the section between your thumb and forefinger, wind and twist the section around the tong until you get to the end of your hair. The twist is very important.

*Try not to wind the section too tightly, you still want to be able to roll the tongs while you are waiting for the curl to set. You also need to be able to slide the tong out from your curl when it has been heated enough.

Let the spring flap close over the tip of the curl and hold the tong until the hair has sufficiently heated. This should take about 15-20 seconds.

Step 7
Release the ends from the tong and slide your hair section out over the tongs without disturbing the curl. Clip the curled section with a pin-curl clip again and leave to cool.

Step 8
Repeat this process with the whole front hairline. If you wish, you can do this over the whole of your head, but it's not necessary.

Step 9
Take out all of the clips and brush the waves into shape (Fig. 2), adjusting the top wave to get the perfect peek-a-boo shape and brushing the ends under and towards your face.

Step 10
Give it all a healthy coating of hairspray to hold.

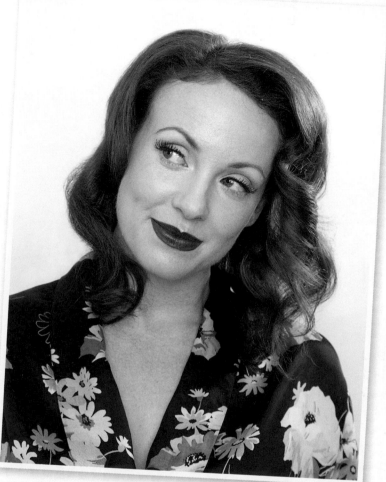

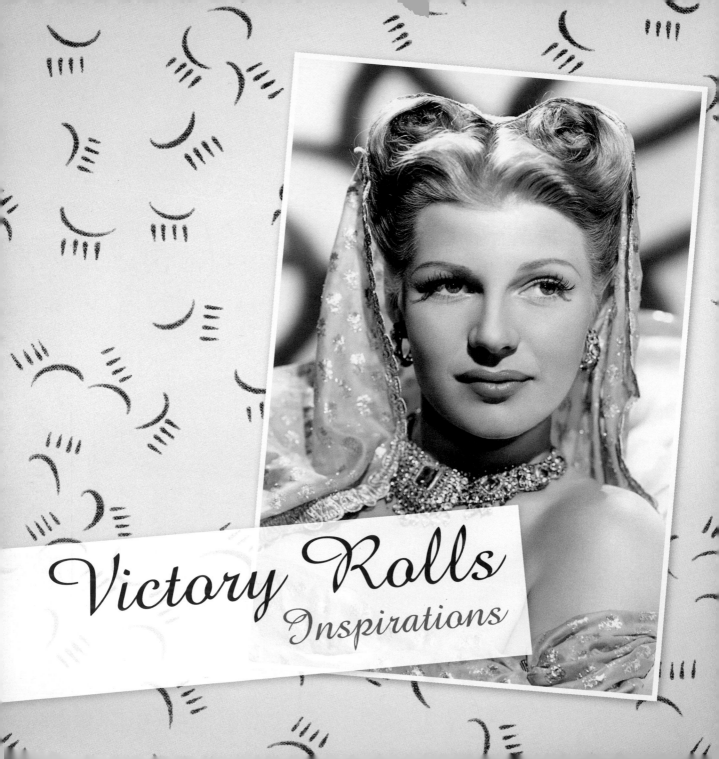

Victory Rolls
Inspirations

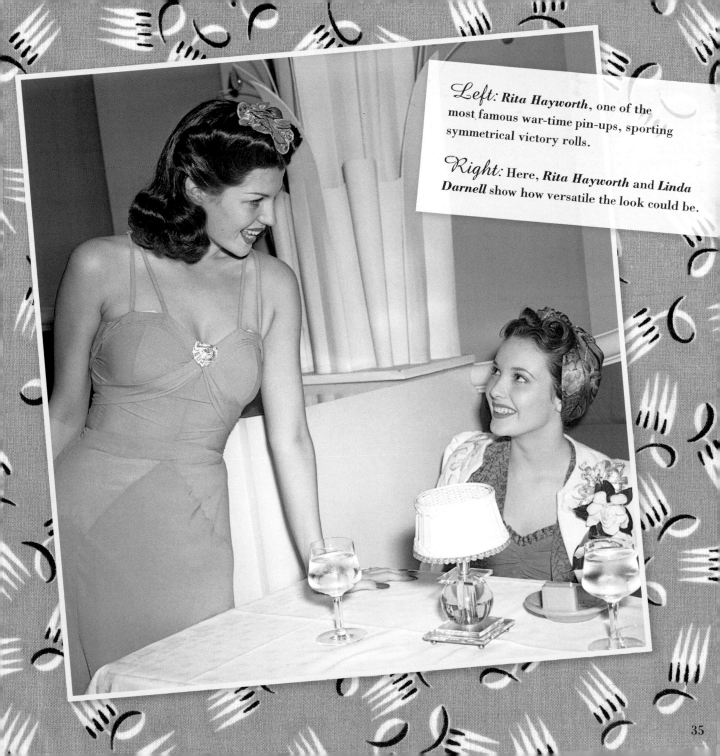

Left: *Rita Hayworth*, one of the most famous war-time pin-ups, sporting symmetrical victory rolls.

Right: Here, *Rita Hayworth* and *Linda Darnell* show how versatile the look could be.

Victory Rolls

The iconic 1940s wartime hairstyle.

In the early 1940s, during World War II, women were rolling up their sleeves and getting involved in the war effort. Fashion was changing due to shortages of fabric and the need to ration. Hairstyles also needed to be practical, as women were being employed to work in factories while their husbands went off to war.

Supposedly named after the manoeuvres of fighter planes, victory rolls were a great way to arrange hair, keeping it safely away from machinery and leaving room to put on a hat without quashing the style!

Modelled at one point by Veronica Lake in a short film encouraging ladies to style their hair in this way, it has become one of our favourite hairstyles to reproduce for a forties revival look.

You will need
Heated rollers *or* hairdryer and pin-curl clips
Combs for backcombing and sectioning
Boar bristle brush for smoothing
Kirby grips
Hairspray

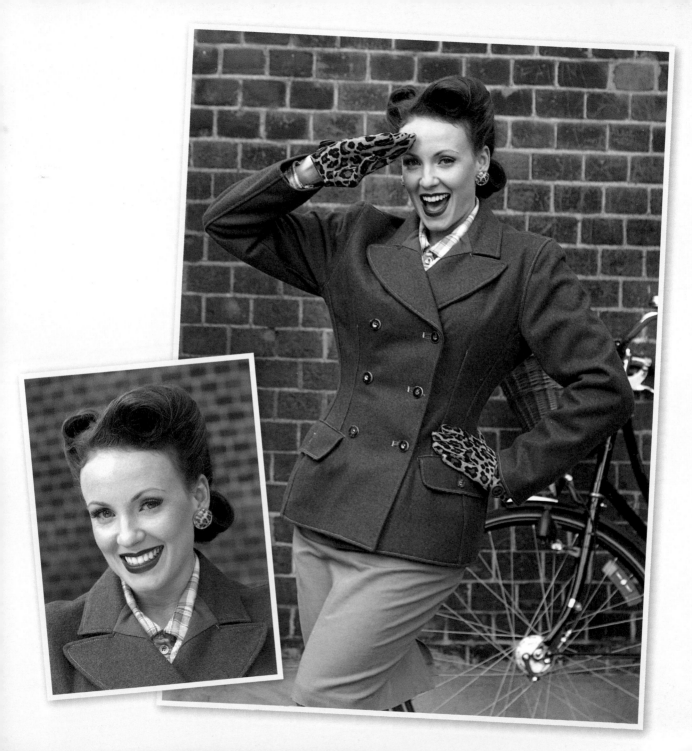

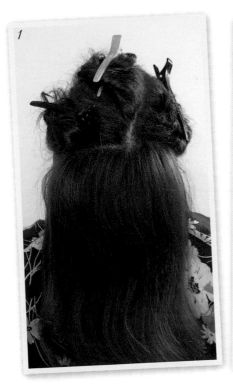

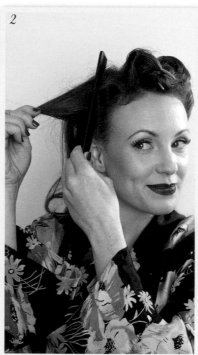

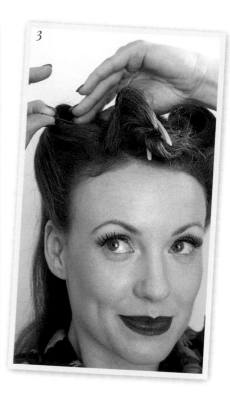

Step 1

Prepare your hair, creating volume using heated rollers or blow drying with a round brush and securing sections with pin-curl clips. Once set, remove your rollers/clips and part your hair on the preferred side.

Step 2

Section and secure your hair into four (Fig.1).

Section 1: your fringe. Take a triangle section from mid-way back on the top of your head to just above both of your temples.

Section 2: left side. Section the whole front part of your hair from the top of your head to the top of your ear.

Section 3: right side, as above.

*One of the sections will probably have more hair in it, because of your side parting.

Section 4: the back of your hair.

Step 3

Backcomb the first side section of your hair for volume and padding. Backcomb taking smaller vertical sections, about 1–2 cm through the larger section (Fig. 2).

Step 4

Roll your hair loosely over your hand, rather like rolling a French pleat. You should be able to hold the finished

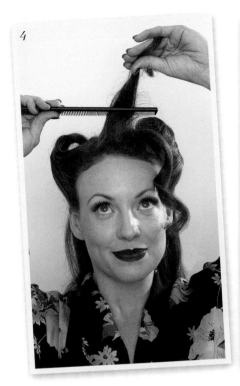

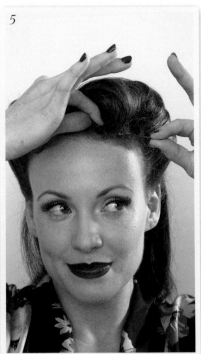

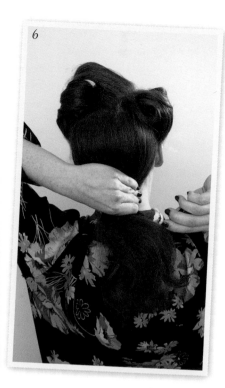

roll securely with one finger so you can see the shape of your victory roll. When you are happy with how it looks, pin it into place and spray with hairspray (Fig. 3). Repeat steps 3 and 4 with the other side section.

Step 5
Backcomb your fringe (Fig. 4). Smooth out the top layer of the backcombing ready to roll it into the rest of the victory rolls.

Step 6
Roll your fringe loosely around your middle three fingers, away from your parting. Try to get the roll the same size

as the largest of your two victory rolls. Pin this into place so that the second roll meets up with your fringe roll (Fig. 5). Now it looks like one roll.

Step 7
Backcomb the back section of your hair for a little extra shape and volume. Smooth over the top layers with your boar bristle brush (Fig. 6).

The beauty of this style is that victory rolls can be created on hair that is bobbed, very long and every length in between.

Step 8

Using Kirby grips, start fixing a row of support grips along your nape (Fig. 7), about 2 cm above your hairline. Each grip should cross over for extra support.

Step 9

Once this has been securely clipped, section the ends of your hair into three parts: the centre and two sides.

Step 10

Backcomb each section very lightly if you need to, smoothing out the underneath layers, as this is the part you will see. Reverse roll each section over your hand and clip into place (Fig. 8).

Your rolls need to be roughly the same size so you can make each section blend together to make one large reverse roll along your back hairline.

Step 11

Spray hair well to smooth down any stray hairs and you have your finished look.

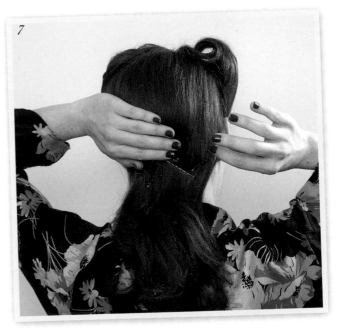

7

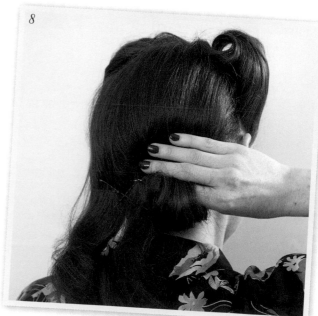

8

Try variations on this style.
Leave the back down and simply curl with tongs.

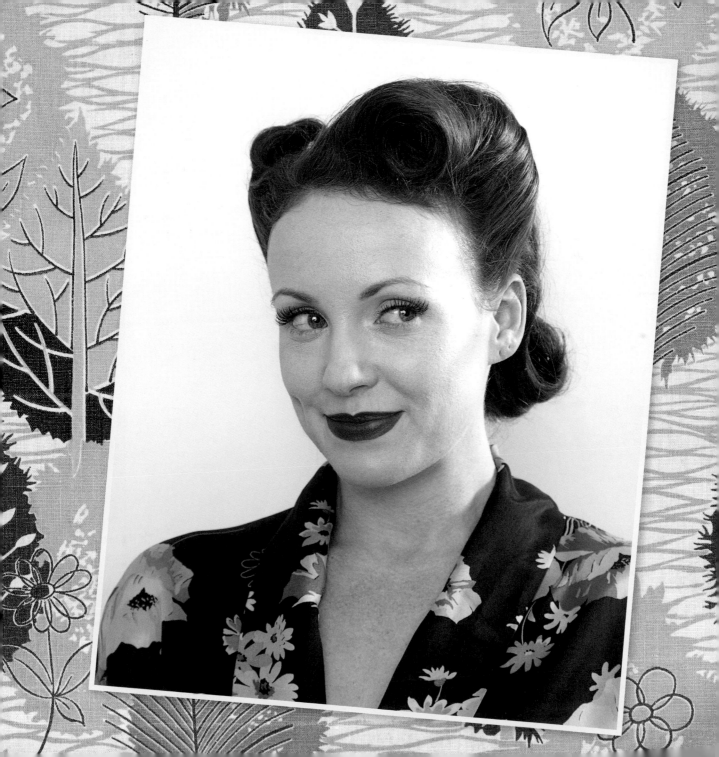

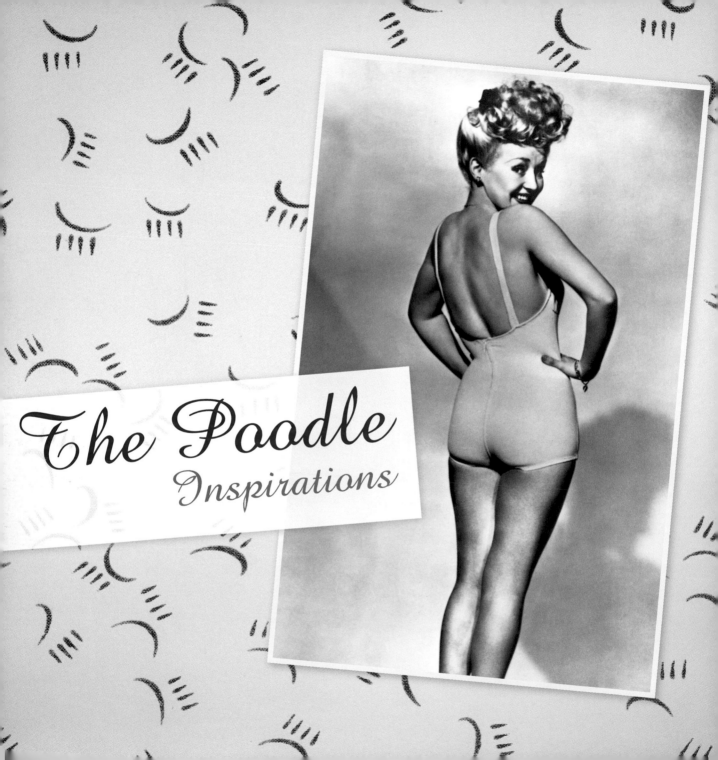

The Poodle
Inspirations

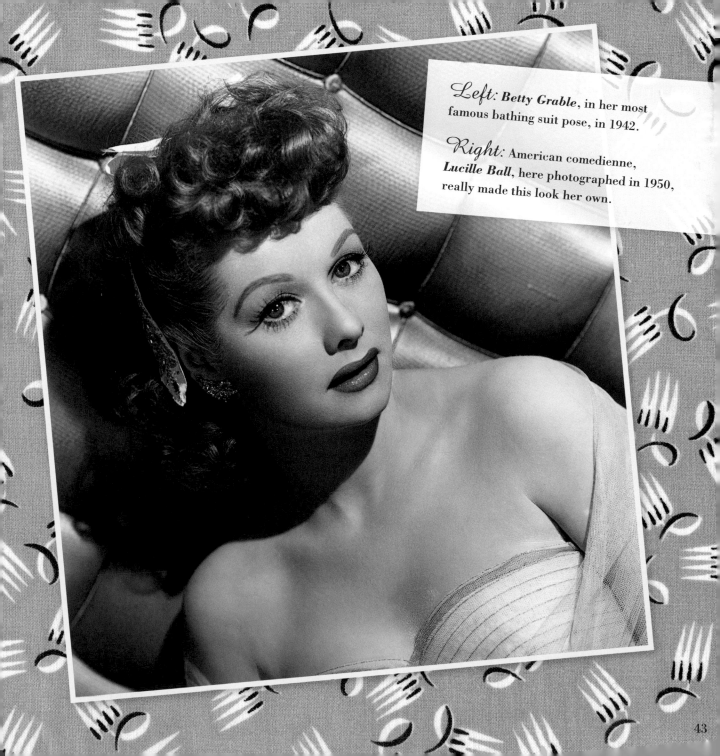

Left: **Betty Grable**, in her most famous bathing suit pose, in 1942.

Right: American comedienne, **Lucille Ball**, here photographed in 1950, really made this look her own.

The Poodle

A popular hairstyle of the forties and fifties, made famous by Lucille Ball and also Betty Grable's iconic 1943 pin-up picture.

In the fifties, curls and soft hairstyles were in! It was considered sophisticated to have curly hair. Fortunately perms had become safer and the results more reliable. So if you were unlucky enough to be a straight-haired girl at this time, you would be off to the hairdresser every six weeks to have a perm. You could even buy a permanent wave kit and try your hand at home. This was an essential part of the hair-care regime for any woman wishing to emulate the poodle and many other styles of the forties and fifties.

This is an interpretation of the fifties Poodle.

You will need
Curling tongs
Hairdryer
Heated rollers, rollers or pin-curl clips
Round brush
Pin-curl clips
Kirby grips and fringe pins
Hairspray

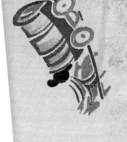
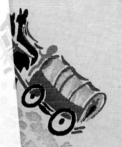
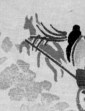
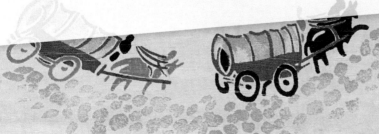

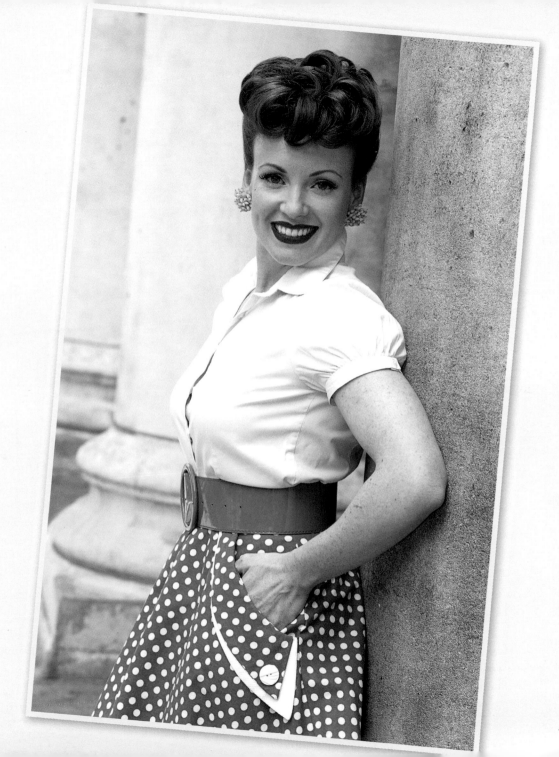

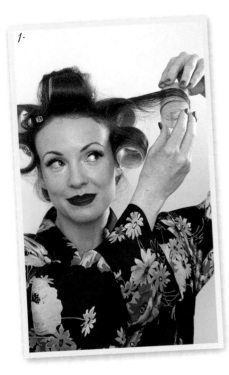

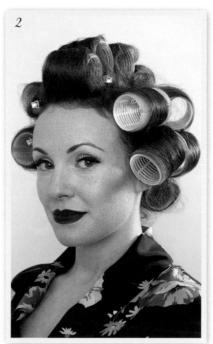

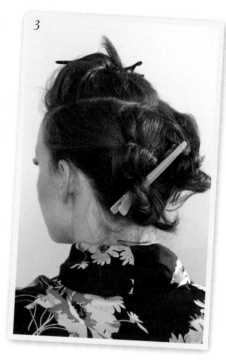

Try using different sized tongs to curl your hair, if you have them. This will give more texture to your curls.

Step 1

Prep your hair to create maximum volume using heated rollers or curling tongs (Figs. 1 and 2). Alternatively, blow dry and secure the hair into curls with pin-curl clips.

Step 2

Spray well with hairspray and leave to cool down for 5–10 minutes.

Step 3

Remove all of your rollers/clips and section your hair into 2 parts (Fig. 3).

Section 1: take a horseshoe-shape section through the top of your head. *This is a curved section from your temple through your crown to your other temple.

Section 2: the rest of your hair (the bottom half). This will be split into 3 later.

Clip the bottom section out of the way.

Step 4

If your hair is still quite straight, use curling tongs to create more curls in the top horseshoe section (Fig. 4).

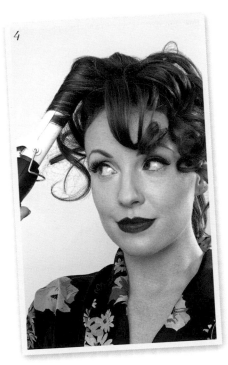

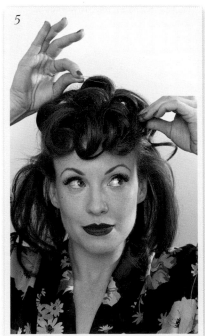

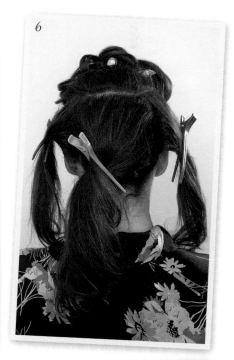

Step 5

Using Kirby grips, start to loosely pin the top into place, making voluminous curls within the section (Fig. 5). Fix these into place with hairspray.

Step 6

Split and clip the bottom section into 3 sections (Fig. 6).
    1: Left side. 2: Right side. 3: Back of your head.

Step 7

Backcomb the sides gently and twist them up to meet the curls in the top section. Secure with grips and leave the ends out to style later (Fig. 7).

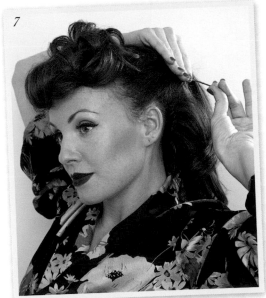

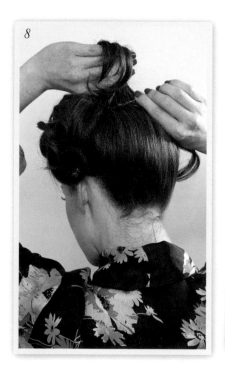

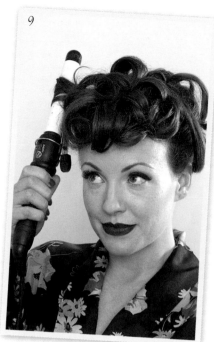

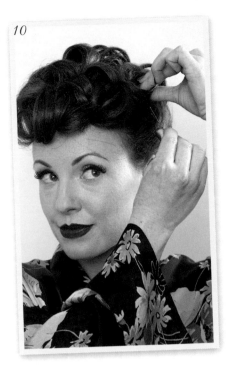

Step 8

Take the back section up to meet the top curly section and, as for the sides, secure with grips (Fig. 8). Again, leave the ends out to curl and secure later.

Step 9

With your curling tongs, curl all of the remaining loose ends (Fig. 9).

Step 10

Arrange all the curls into shape, secure with grips (Fig. 10) and give a final spray with hairspray to hold.

This style looks adorable wrapped up in a 1940s-style scarf (see pages 102–103).

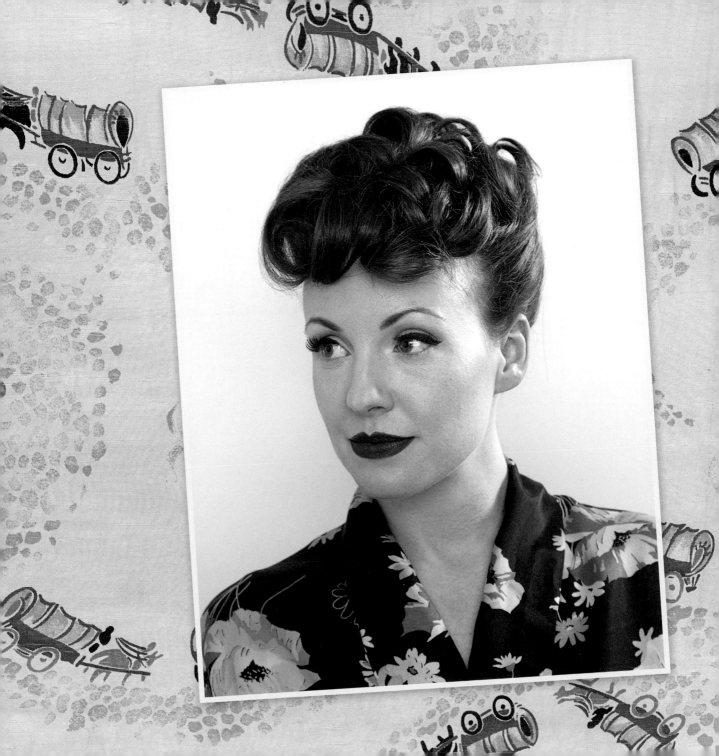

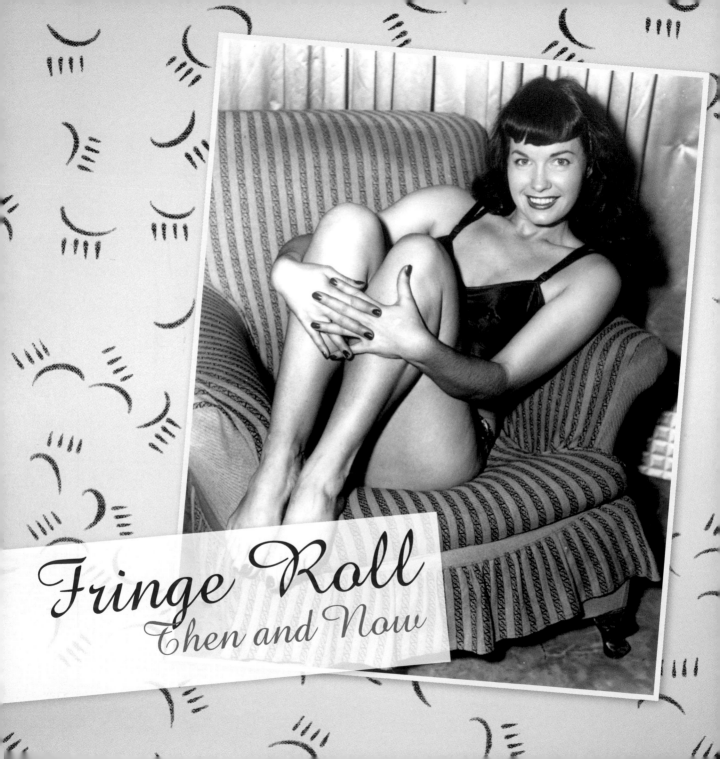

Fringe Roll
Then and Now

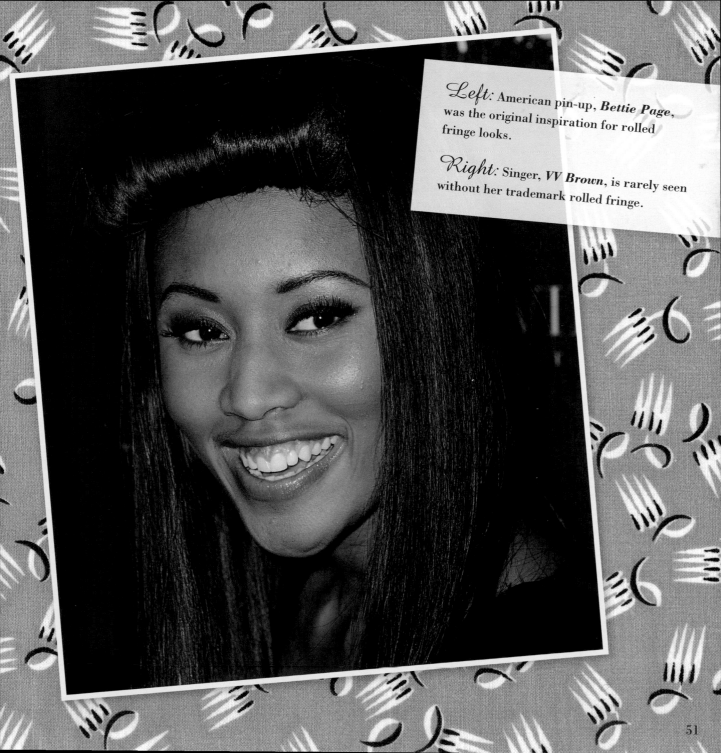

Left: American pin-up, *Bettie Page*, was the original inspiration for rolled fringe looks.

Right: Singer, *VV Brown*, is rarely seen without her trademark rolled fringe.

The VV Forward Fringe Roll

This style is ideal for anyone who doesn't have a fringe.

The fringe roll is an adaptation of the Bettie Page fringe. Bettie Page was the notorious pin-up girl made famous in the fifties by posing for Hugh Hefner. Never quite as mainstream as Marilyn, she nevertheless developed a cult following and later in life was even the subject of a motion picture. The rolled fringe was fashioned by girls so they could emulate Bettie's trademark fringe without having to commit to a full fringe cut.

The rolled fringe can also be used in conjunction with victory rolls.

You will need
Kirby grips
Hair padding (roly poly)
Hair ties
Curling tongs
Combs
Hairspray

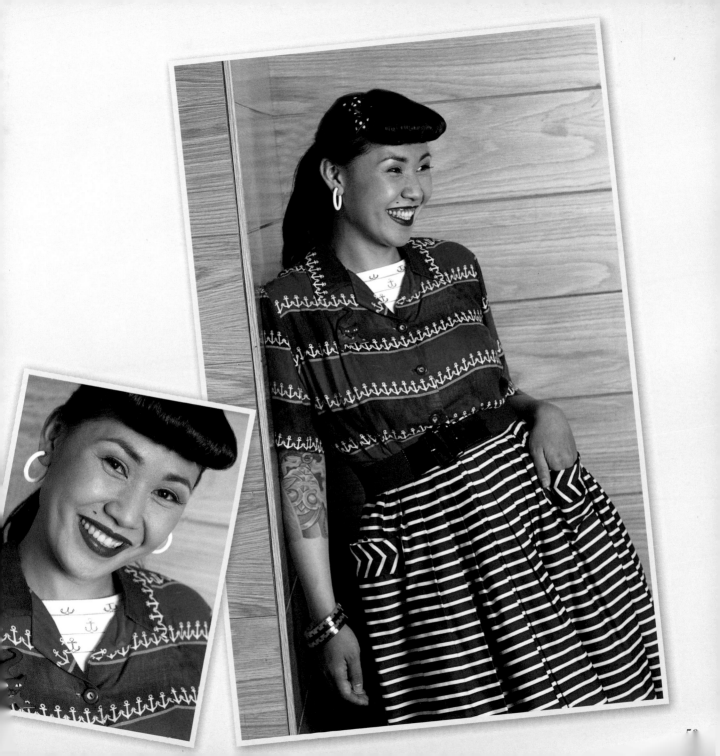

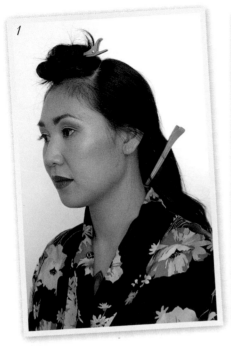

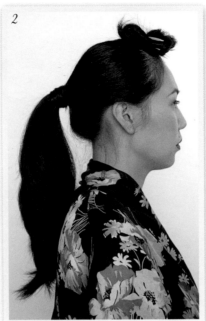

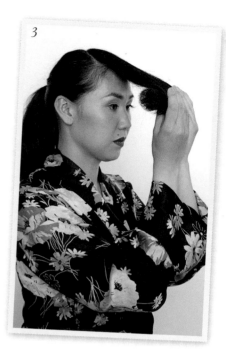

Step 1

Take a small triangle section at the front of your head from the recessions of your front hairline (this is usually where your hairline starts to curve around towards your temples). Secure it out of the way (Fig. 1).

Step 2

Secure the rest of your hair into a ponytail (Fig. 2).

It looks super cute, if you have straight hair, to curl your ponytail using curling tongs.

Step 3

Removing the clip from your front section, take small sections and backcomb to give height and body. This will also make your hairstyle more stable.

Step 4

Smooth out your backcombing and take a small roly poly hair pad (you can find these in chemists or hairdressing suppliers). It needs to be the shape of a sausage or banana.

Roll the ends of your fringe over and around the hair pad, keeping tension from the roots of your hair as you go (Fig. 3).

Step 5

Secure the roll with grips on either side of your head and spread your hair around the padding to hide it (Fig. 4).

Step 6

Spray with hairspray to hold.

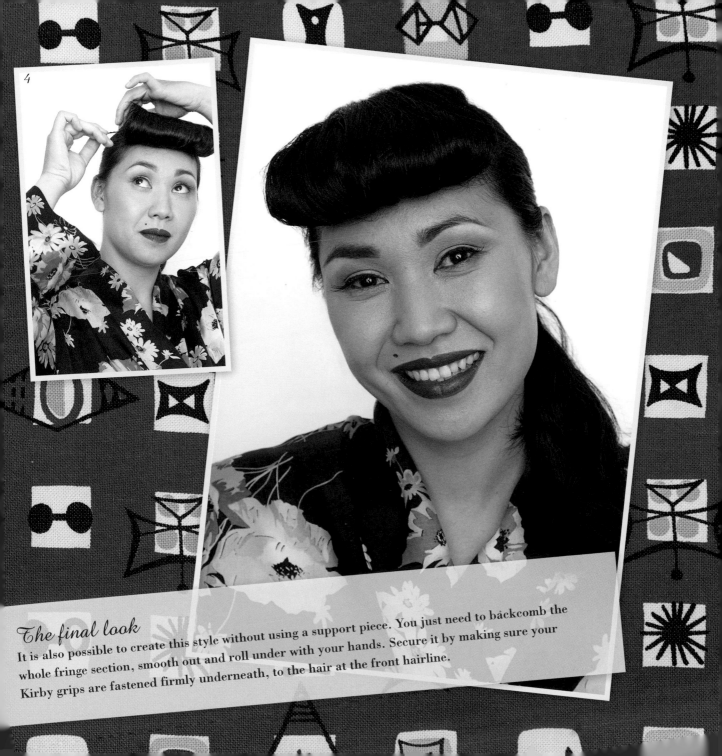

4

The final look

It is also possible to create this style without using a support piece. You just need to backcomb the whole fringe section, smooth out and roll under with your hands. Secure it by making sure your Kirby grips are fastened firmly underneath, to the hair at the front hairline.

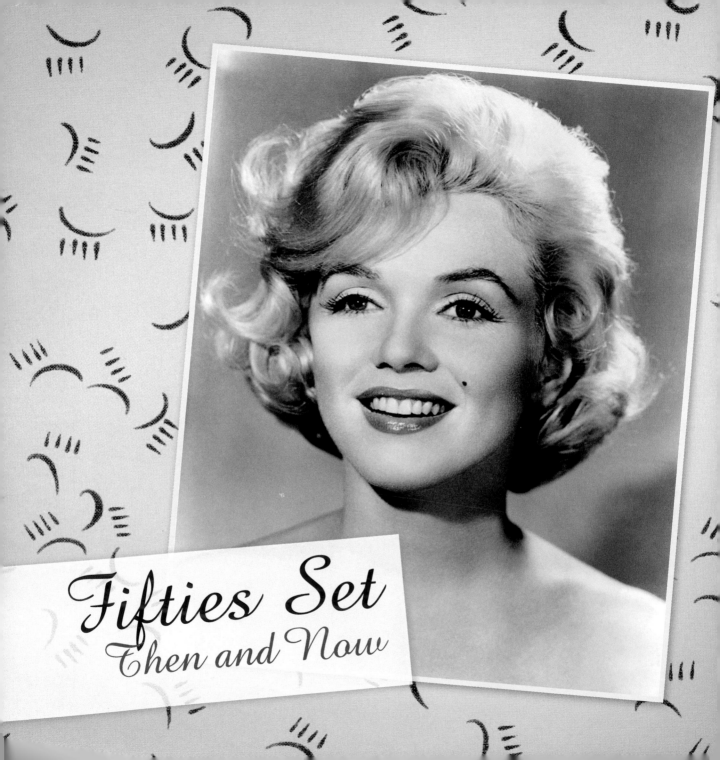

Fifties Set
Then and Now

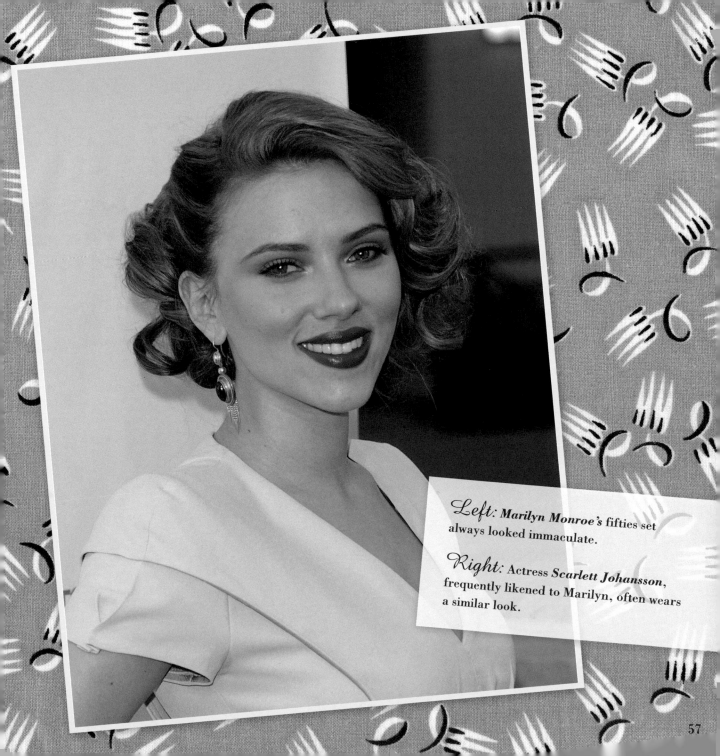

Left: **Marilyn Monroe's** fifties set always looked immaculate.

Right: Actress **Scarlett Johansson**, frequently likened to Marilyn, often wears a similar look.

The Marilyn Set

Women in the forties and fifties would spend hours styling their hair. It was usual to make regular weekly trips to the hairdresser for a shampoo and set. During the war, when money was tight, the weekly trips may have become fortnightly trips – this is when tying scarves came in very handy. Women would also have their own set of rollers and learned to roll up and pin curl their own hair at home. It wasn't unusual for women to spend all day working around the house with rollers in, setting their hair ready for their evening out.

You will need
Rollers and pins
Pin-tail comb
Portable dryer
Styling products

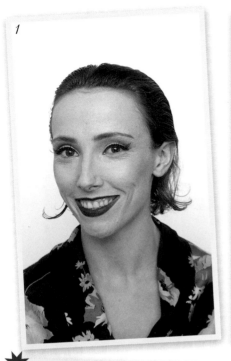

1

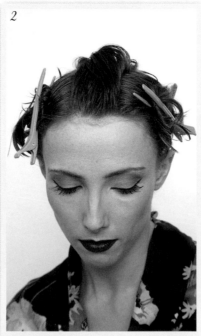

2

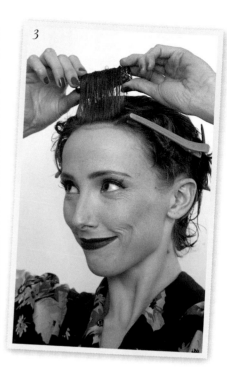

3

Step 1

Shampoo and towel dry your hair. Apply mousse, setting lotion or other styling products and comb though (Fig. 1).

Step 2

Section your hair into 5 (Fig. 2).

Section 1: a section, the width of your roller, directly over the centre of your head – from your front hairline to back hairline.

Section 2: a roller width down and through the front left side of your head.

Section 3: a roller width down and through the back left side of your head.

Section 4: a roller width down and through the front right side of your head.

Section 5: a roller width down and through the back right side of your head.

Secure all the sections out of the way.

Step 3

Start working on the first section of hair – the section that runs over the centre of your head.

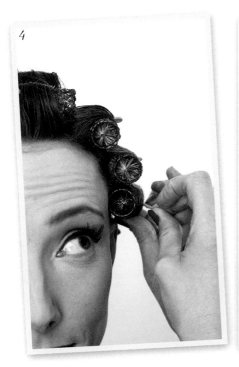

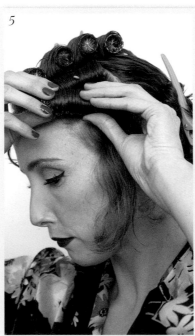

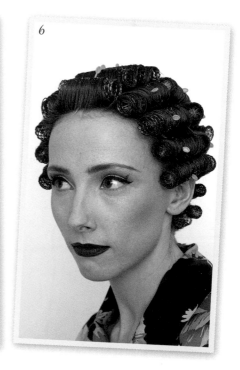

Take a 2 cm section of hair horizontally across the front of the section. Comb this section straight up from your head. Hold the ends of the section between your thumb and index finger.

With the other hand place a roller at the end of your section and flip the ends of the hair over the top of the roller (Fig. 3).

Roll this up, use the end of a pintail comb to drag the ends under to the centre of the roller, so you don't get fishhooks (pieces of hair that are folded sharply in the wrong direction), as they make the ends of your hair look fluffy. Fix in place (Fig. 4).

Step 4
Continue this all the way through the centre section. You may need someone to help you with the back.

Step 5
Start rolling up the sides in the same way (Fig. 5). Each of the sections needs to be combed directly out from your head so the rollers are rolled on the base of your hair (the hair is directed straight out from the head once the roller is secure).

Step 6
Continue this for the entire head (see Figs. 6 and 7 for ideal placement of rollers).

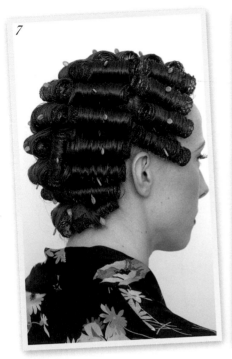

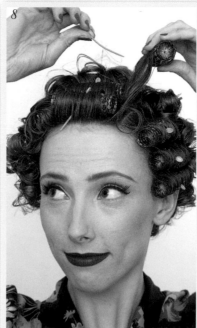

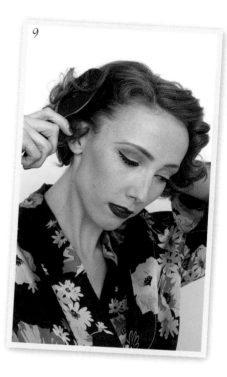

Step 7

Once your hair has been completely rolled up into the set, you can either sit under a portable dryer (which should take about 30 minutes) or leave it to dry naturally (which could take 8–12 hours depending on the thickness of your hair).

Step 8

Remove all of the rollers once your hair is completely dry (Fig. 8).

Step 9

Using a boar bristle brush, start to brush out your curls (Fig. 9). You can be quite firm while brushing them out. Work the ends under with the brush and turn them inwards towards your face.

Step 10

Spray with hairspray to hold.

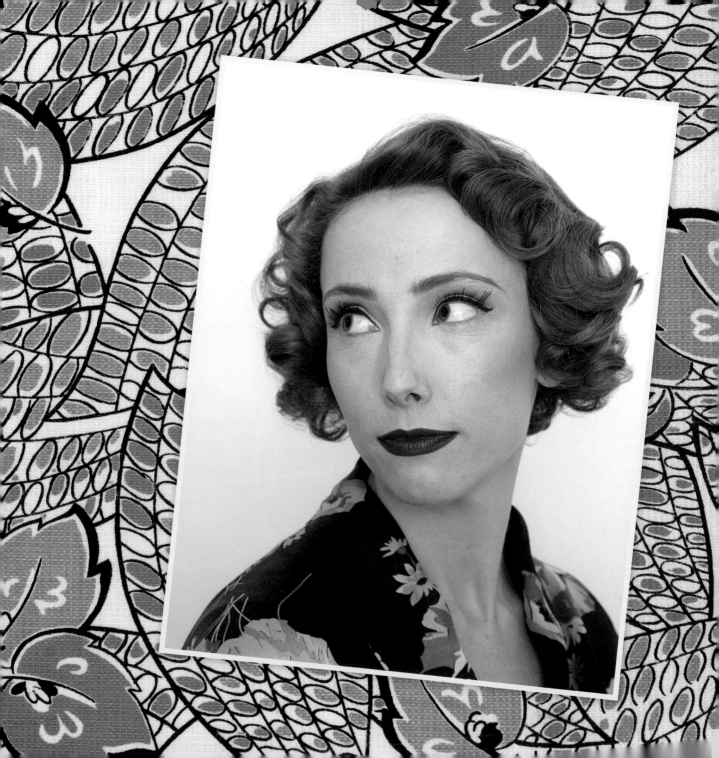

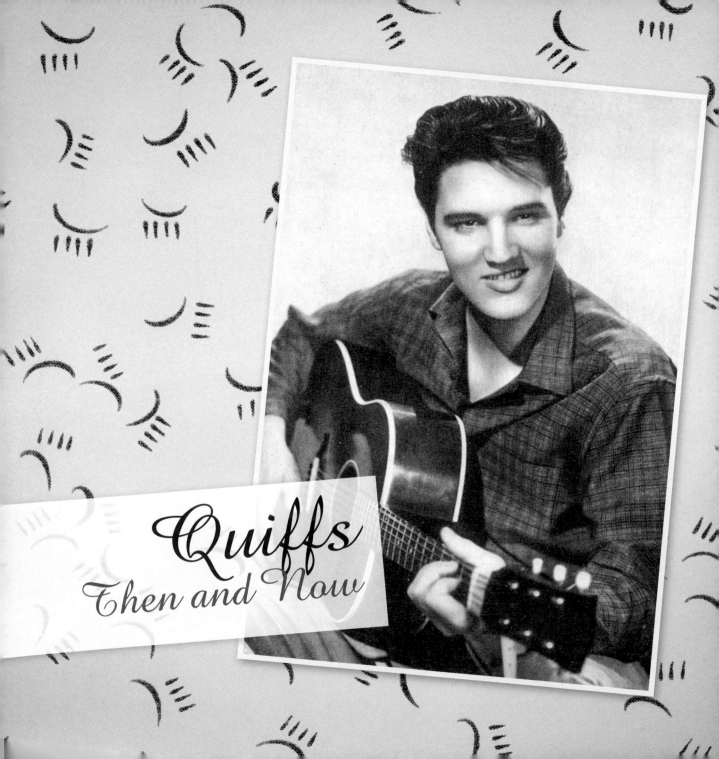

Quiffs
Then and Now

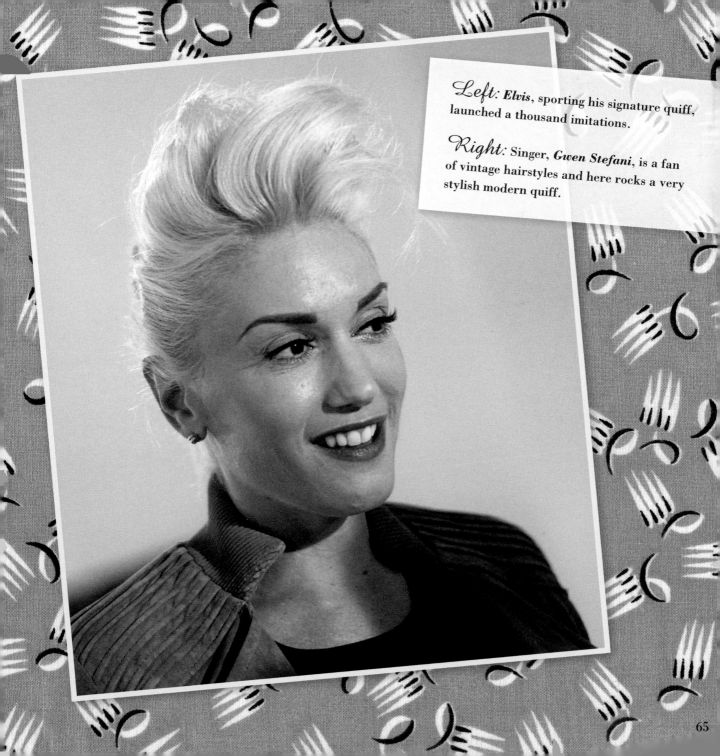

Left: *Elvis*, sporting his signature quiff, launched a thousand imitations.

Right: Singer, *Gwen Stefani*, is a fan of vintage hairstyles and here rocks a very stylish modern quiff.

The Pompadour (Quiff)

This is a straightforward way to achieve a classic and fun fifties look.

The quiff or pompadour was a popular style in the fifties among the rockabilly guys. It was made famous by James Dean and years later by John Travolta in *Grease*, but was actually named after Madam de Pompadour, the chief mistress of King Louis XV of France.

This style has become a favourite with today's rockabilly girls because of its obvious nod to the fifties and the fact that it can usually be worn with a ponytail, which is great to swing and flip around while dancing!

Remember – there are many ways to style a pompadour. You can roll it different ways or wear it scruffy, depending on the length or your hair.

Alas! If you have a short fringe, you may have to grow it a bit to be able to quiff it. For this style you need to have a reasonably long fringe or no fringe at all.

You will need
Kirby grips
Comb
Hairspray
Ponytail elastic
Curling tongs

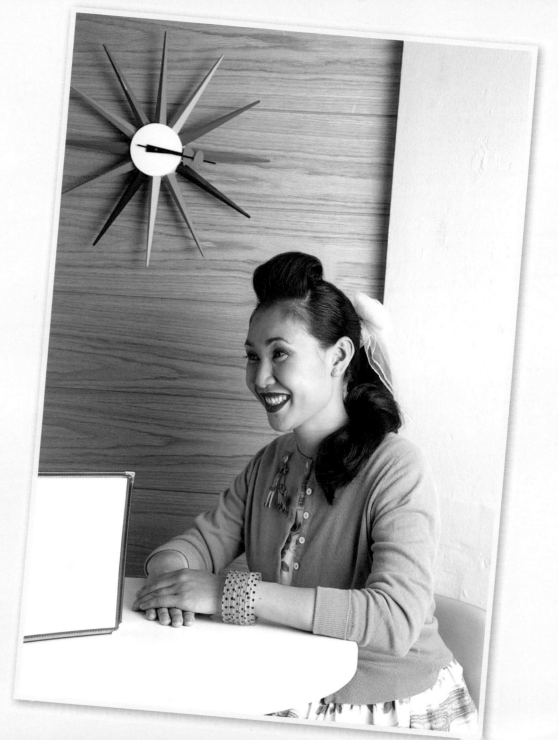

Step 1

Take a small triangle section at the front of your head from the recessions of your front hairline (this is usually where your hairline starts to curve around towards your temples). Secure it out of the way.

Step 2

Secure the rest of your hair into a ponytail.

It looks super cute, if you have straight hair, to curl your ponytail using curling tongs.

Step 3

Remove the clip from your front section. Take small sections and backcomb to give height and body. This will also make your hairstyle more stable.

Step 4

Smooth the front of the section out with a boar bristle brush and start to roll your hair around your 3 middle fingers. If you want a larger or smaller quiff use more or less fingers to roll your hair (Fig. 1).

*If you want a more modern quiff, you don't need to smooth out the backcombing.

Step 5

Use your finger as a makeshift Kirby grip before you secure the grip directly under your finger (Fig. 2). You may need to use a few grips to make sure it stays in place.

Step 6

Spray well with hairspray to hold.

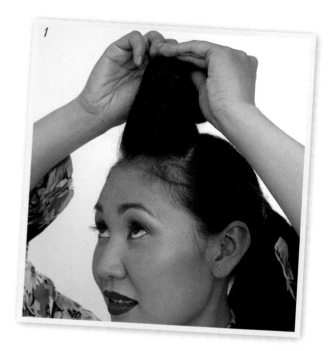

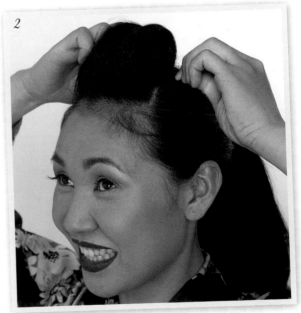

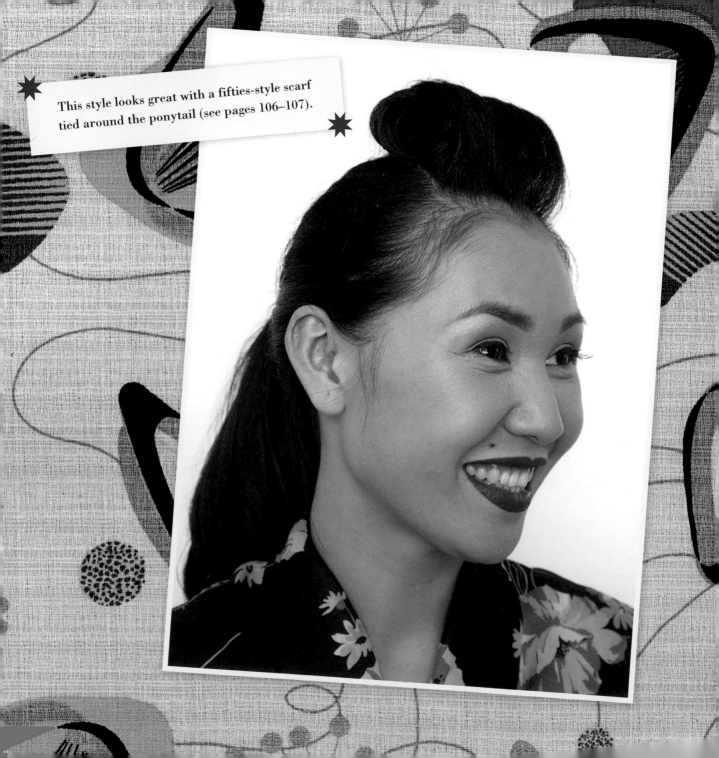

This style looks great with a fifties-style scarf tied around the ponytail (see pages 106–107).

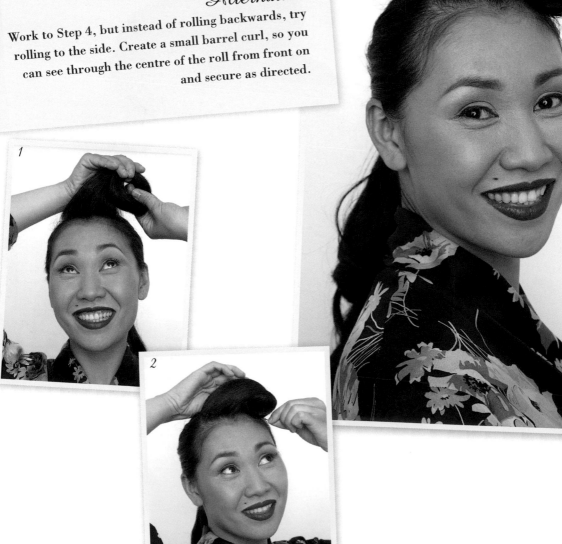

Work to Step 4, but instead of rolling backwards, try rolling to the side. Create a small barrel curl, so you can see through the centre of the roll from front on and secure as directed.

1

2

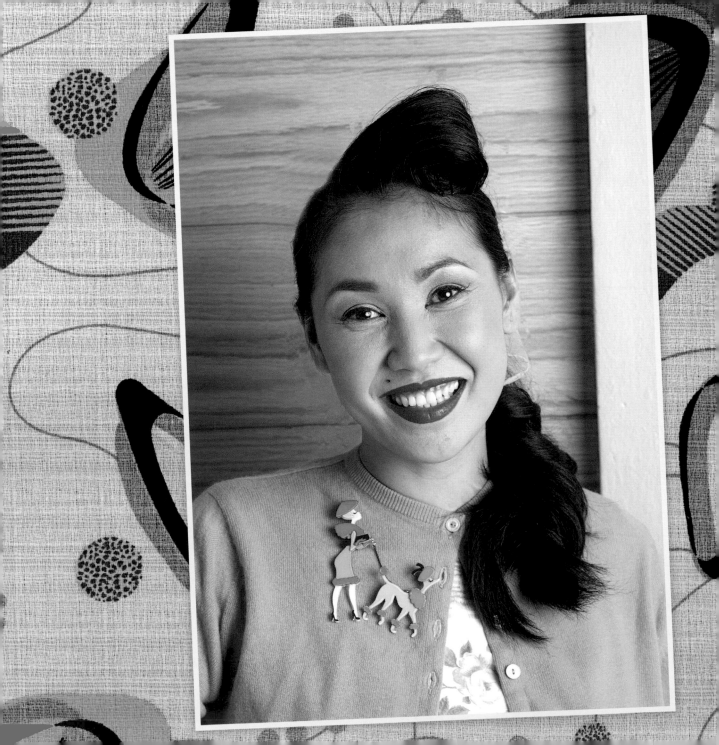

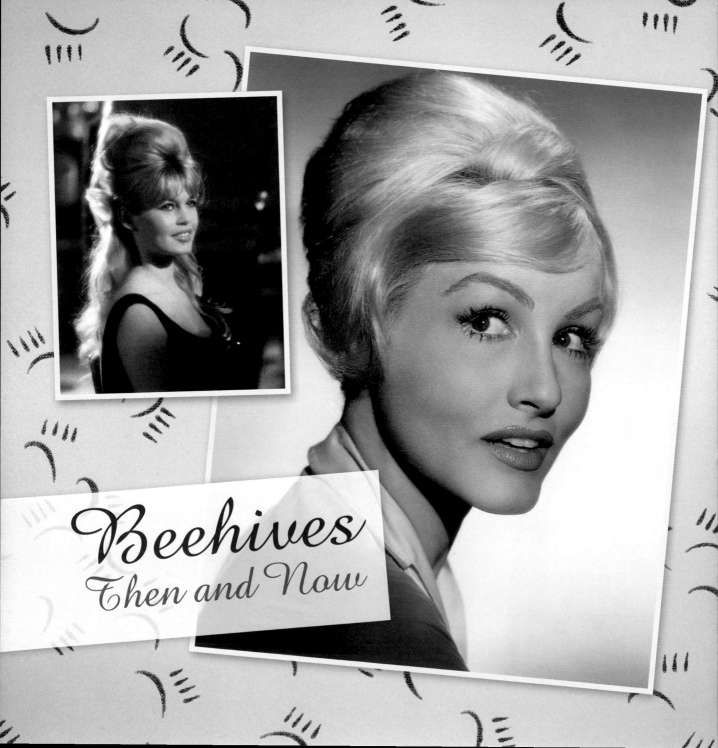

Beehives
Then and Now

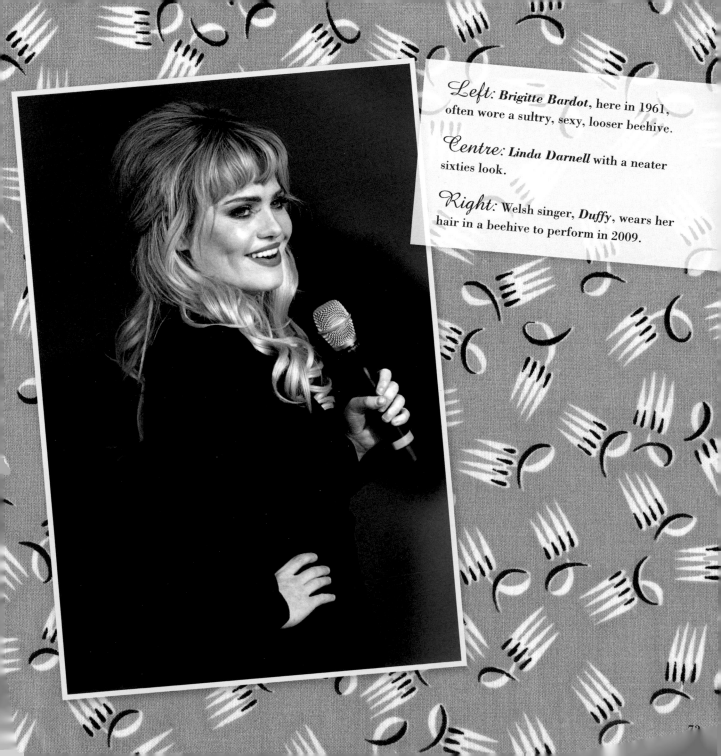

Left: *Brigitte Bardot*, here in 1961, often wore a sultry, sexy, looser beehive.

Centre: *Linda Darnell* with a neater sixties look.

Right: Welsh singer, *Duffy*, wears her hair in a beehive to perform in 2009.

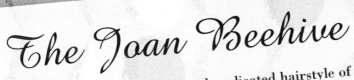

The Joan Beehive

The beehive was the most sought-after and replicated hairstyle of the 1960s and is still iconic of that time, along with the Beatles and the mini skirt. Given its name because of its similarity to the shape of old-fashioned beehives, it remains a popular hairstyle for weddings and social events, on the catwalk, and even as an every-day style for some.

In this book we have included two different styles of beehive, because there are so many different ways you can create this look. The first (The Joan) is created using padding, which gives extra height and volume to your hair. If you have fine hair this is the easiest version to try to help you create a huge beehive.

See page 80 for the second beehive variation.

You will need
Hairdryer
Round brush
Pin-curl clips, heated rollers or curling tongs
Comb
Section clips
Soft bristle brush for smoothing
Kirby grips
Hair padding

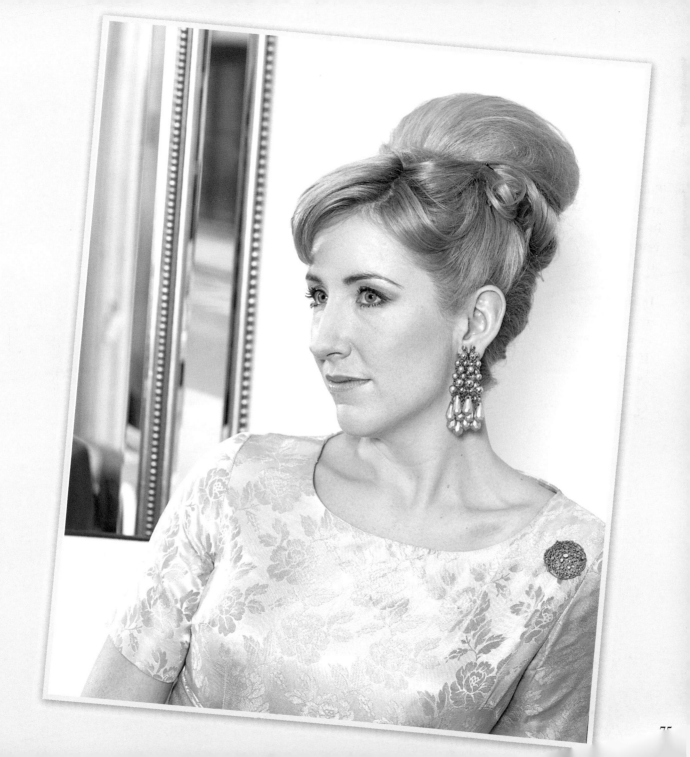

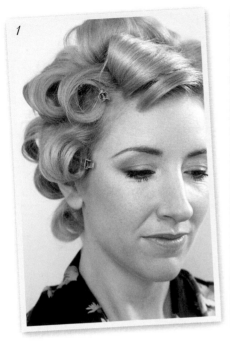

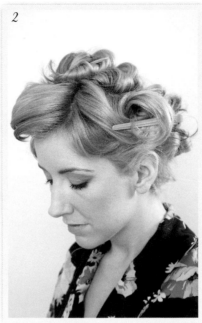

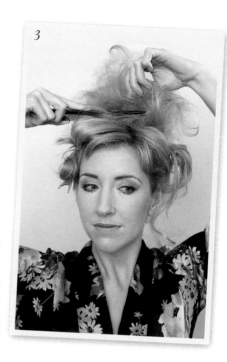

Step 1

Prep your hair to get volume and wave, using heated rollers, tongs or a hair dryer and pin-curl clips (Fig. 1).

Step 2

Section your hair into five parts (Fig. 2).

Section 1: the fringe.

Section 2: the top of your head to below the crown.

Section 3: the left side of your head roughly 2 cm behind your ear.

Section 4: the right side of your head roughly 2 cm behind your ear (both the left and right side are put up in the same way so will be dealt with together).

Section 5: the back of your head.

Clip all of the sections neatly away.

Step 3

Unclip the section at the top of your head and start taking smaller sections through it. Backcomb each of these small sections from the front to the back, using hairspray between sections, until the entire top section has been backcombed (Fig. 3).

* Don't be afraid to make this as big as you can. You can make it smaller when you start to secure the shape.

Step 4

Secure your hair padding into place around the crown area using Kirby grips (Fig. 4).

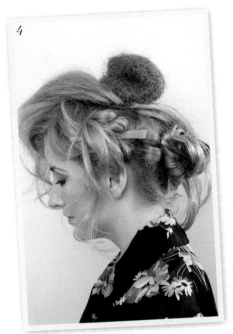
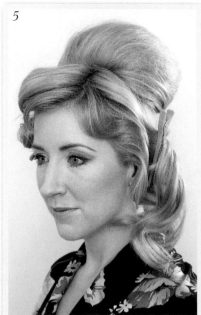
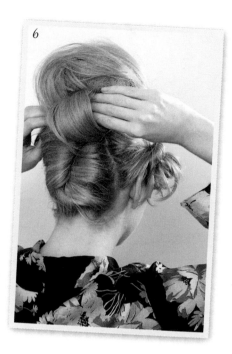

Step 5

Start covering the hair padding with your backcombed sections of hair, smoothing out your sections with a soft boar bristle brush as you go along (Fig. 5). Be careful not to completely brush out your backcombing.

Play around until you are happy with the shape and height of the hair that is covering the padding.

Step 6

Take the section at the back of your head and start backcombing in smaller vertical sections.

Smooth the top layer of this section and twist this hair into a French pleat leaving the ends out to style later (Fig. 6). Secure with Kirby grips.

Step 7

Secure the ends of the French pleat in a barrel curl under the hair pad with Kirby grips (Figs. 7a and 7b).

Step 8

If you have fine hair you may want to gently backcomb the sides taking sections running vertically along your head from back to front.

Smooth the sides up to where your hair padding has been placed and covered, and secure with Kirby grips, leaving the ends out to style later (Fig. 8).

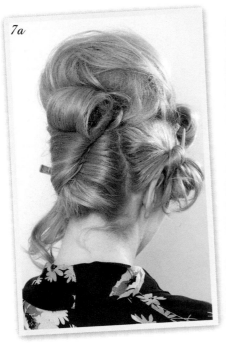

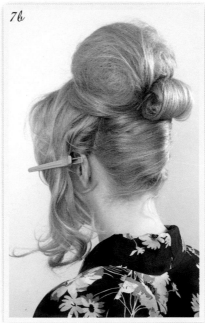

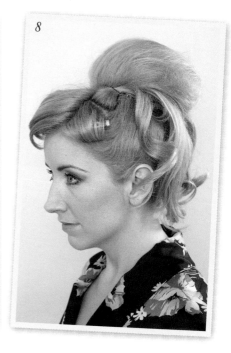

Step 9

The ends of your hair now need to be styled and pinned. Secure these ends in barrel-type curls around the hair pad (Fig. 9). Be patient, sometimes this takes a bit of time.

Step 10

Release the fringe from its clip and backcomb for volume. Smooth over the layer and comb in the desired direction.

Step 11

Spray your hair with hairspray to keep it all smooth and in place.

REMEMBER!
You are probably a few inches taller now. Be careful, when you are gracefully sliding into your taxi or limo, that you don't knock your beehive out of shape.

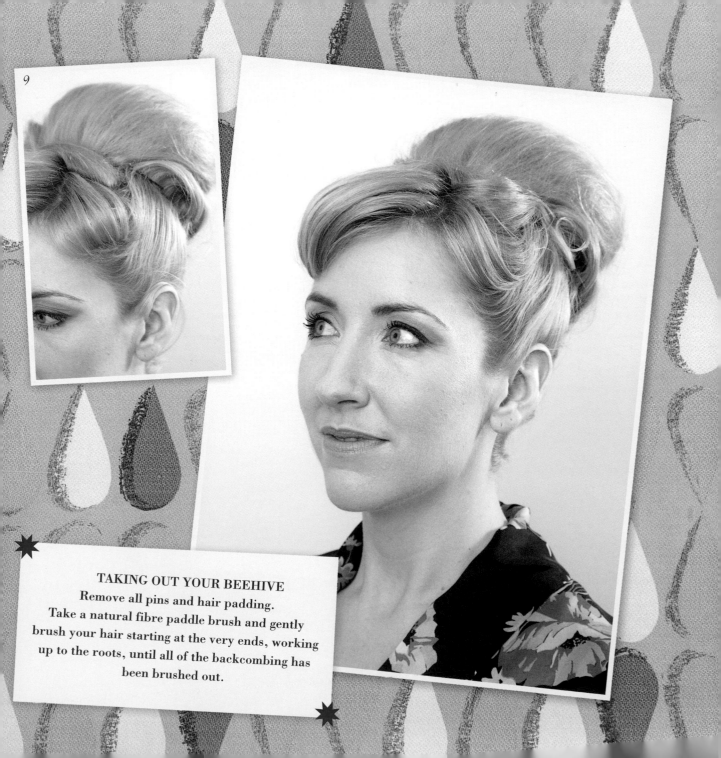

9

TAKING OUT YOUR BEEHIVE
Remove all pins and hair padding.
Take a natural fibre paddle brush and gently
brush your hair starting at the very ends, working
up to the roots, until all of the backcombing has
been brushed out.

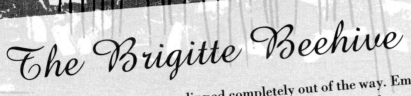

The Brigitte Beehive

The hair in a beehive wasn't always clipped completely out of the way. Emerging from the bouffant hairstyle, it also became popular for beehives to have a little bit of hair left down. Usually worn curly, this sexy style was seen on Brigitte Bardot and copied by countless fans in the sixties.

This is a softer beehive, fashioned without using a hairpiece. It is created with backcombing, which is a quicker and easier way to build a beehive, and better for thicker hair.

For a more modern style, you can backcomb your hair and smooth it just enough to give you shape, leaving you with a messy, textured beehive.

You will need
Rollers
Curling tongs
Hair ties
Comb
Hairspray
Boar bristle brush
Kirby grips

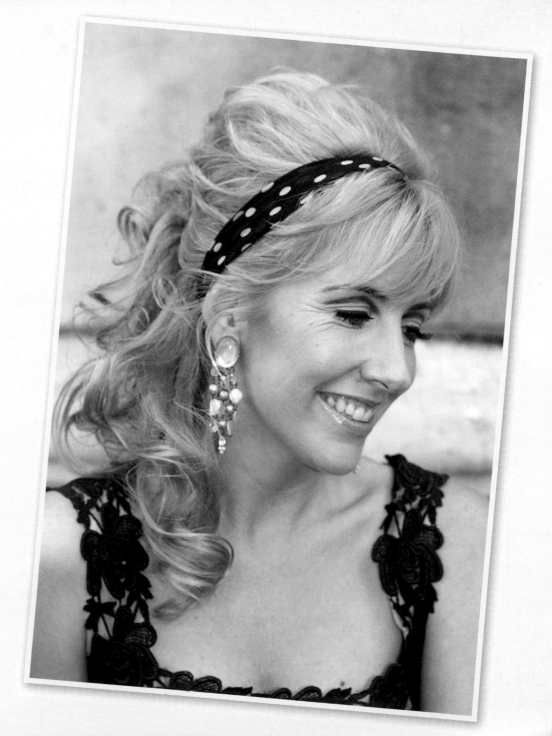

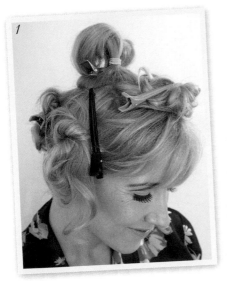
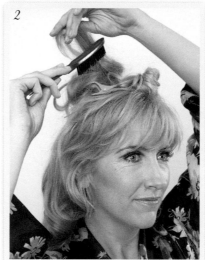
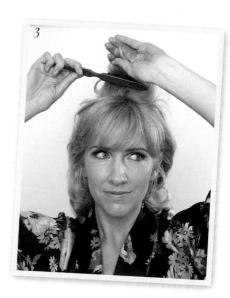

Step 1

Prep your hair using rollers or tongs for volume and wave.

Step 2

Take a diamond section of hair around your crown and tie it into a ponytail (Fig. 1). Section off the top, sides and back of the hair and clip away.

Step 3

Split the ponytail into smaller sections and start backcombing each section to create volume (Fig. 2).

Fasten the sections around the ponytail with Kirby grips to create the padding for your beehive.

Step 4

Separate the top of your hair from the sides and start to backcomb, taking sections diagonally across your head (Fig. 3). Spray with hairspray from time to time to hold.

Step 5

Smooth this section over the top of the backcombed ponytail. You can do this by rolling the section loosely over your hand and pinning the section below the ponytail with Kirby grips. Arrange the height at the top into shape and spray with hairspray to hold.

Step 6

Backcomb the sides in the same way as the top section. Smooth and pin them into place by rolling them inwards around your fingers towards the ponytail (Fig. 4). The ends from the top and sides should be tucked away, covering the original ponytail (Fig. 5). Spray with hairspray.

Step 7

Tong the ends of your hair if you prefer curly ends (this hairstyle could also look great with straight ends, if you prefer this, you could stop here).

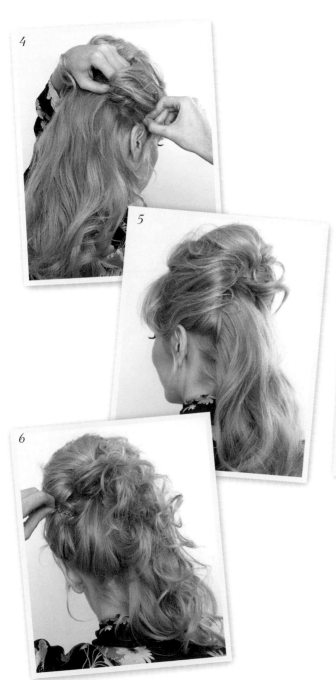

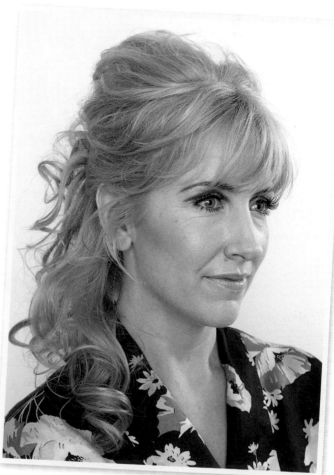

Step 8

Pin the curled ends loosely up towards the ponytail to create a tousled look (Fig. 6). Spray with hairspray to hold.

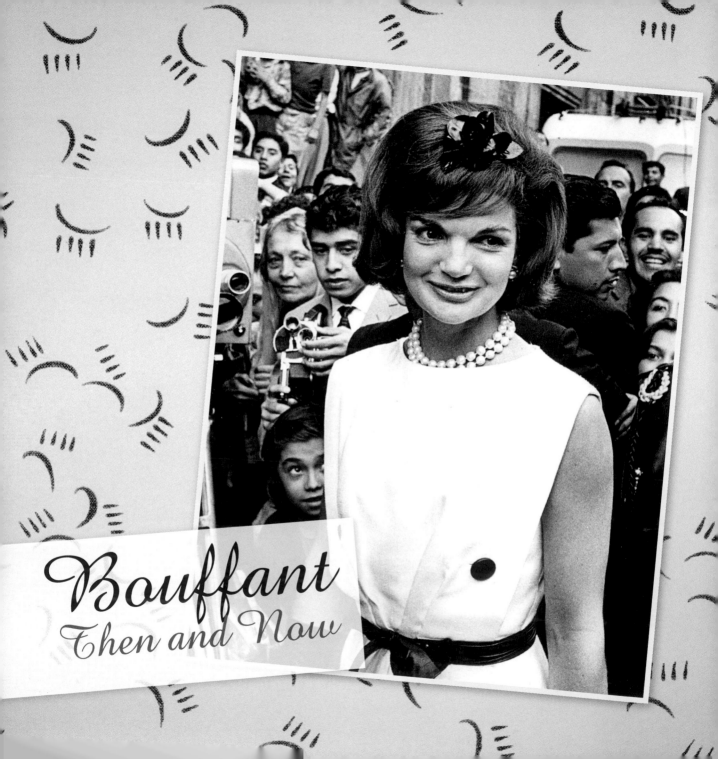

Bouffant
Then and Now

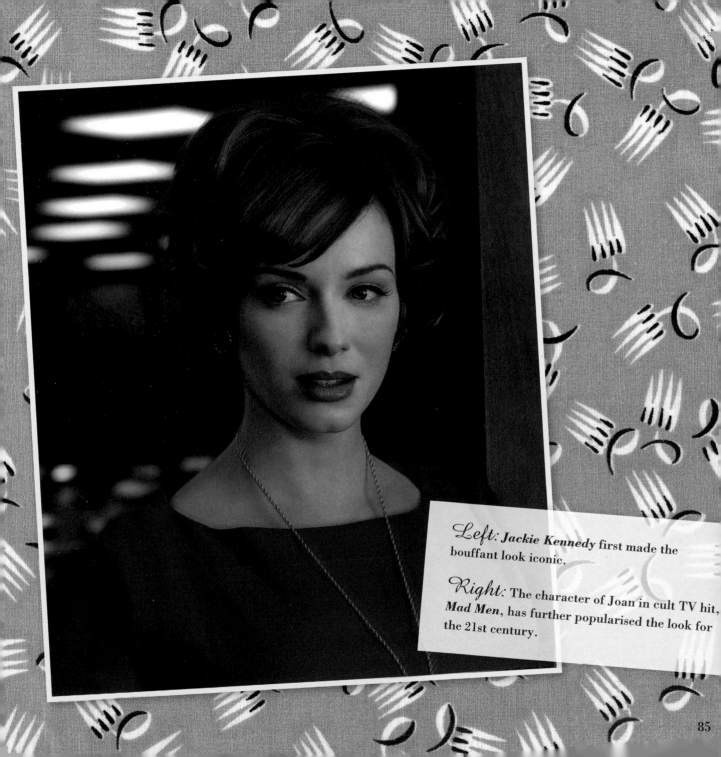

*Left: **Jackie Kennedy** first made the bouffant look iconic.*

*Right: The character of Joan in cult TV hit, **Mad Men**, has further popularised the look for the 21st century.*

The Jackie O Bouffant

Although this hairstyle is an icon of the sixties, it actually came into fashion in the fifties in the United States; the UK followed suit a few years later. It was designed to balance out the full-skirted shape of fifties dresses.

There was a lot of debate among fashion journalists and hairstylists in the fifties as to whether the bouffant would remain in style for long. People were concerned that it might be unflattering to their face shape and later that it was actually unhealthy to backcomb the hair so much. But Jackie Kennedy finally gave it iconic status in 1960 and it was here to stay, remaining in fashion until the end of the sixties.

The bouffant style took many different forms, it was a catch-all term for hair that was oversized and loosely coiffed.

You will need
Curling tongs
Comb
Pin tail comb
Rollers
Hairspray

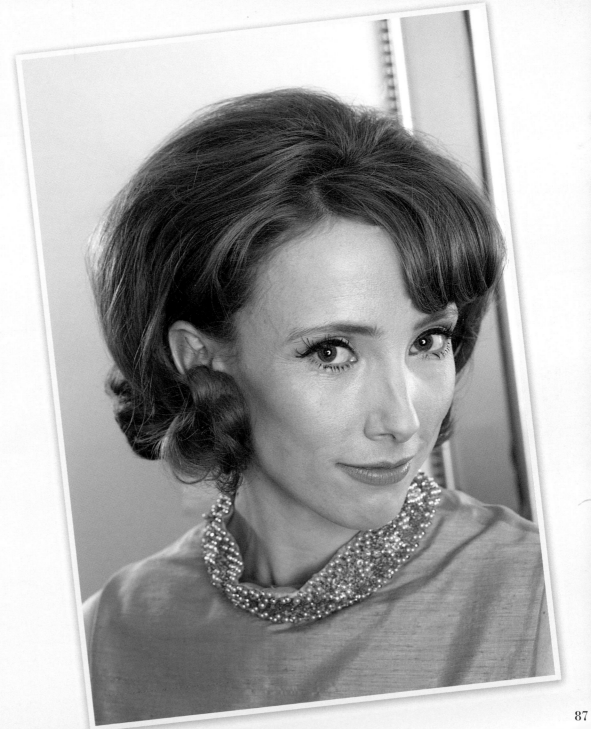

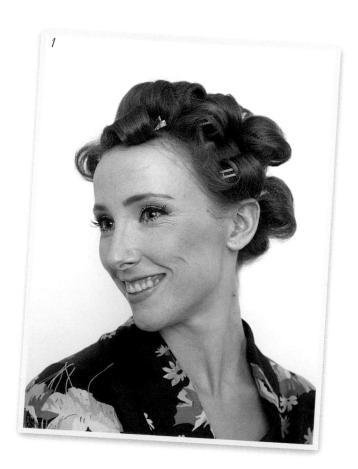

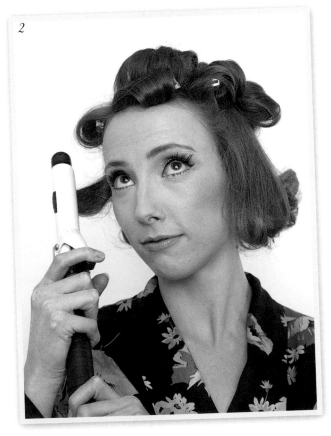

Step 1

Prep your hair to create volume using heated rollers, curling tongs, or a hair dryer and pin curl clips (Fig. 1).

Step 2

Remove the rollers/clips from the curled sections around the bottom of your hairline. Start to tong these sections in reverse (away from your face) so your hair will flick up (Fig. 2).

Step 3

Backcomb this underneath section at the roots to give some root lift and smooth out.

Step 4

Remove the rest of your rollers and take a section through the middle of your head to just below the crown and start to backcomb the hair (Fig. 3). Make the hair as big as possible. Spray with hairspray to fix.

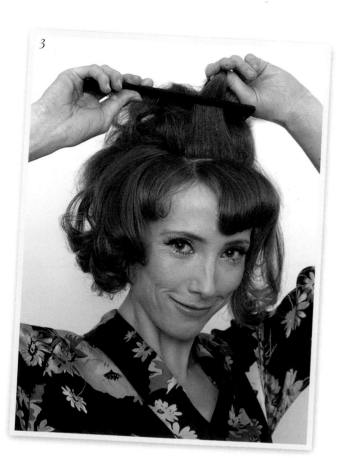

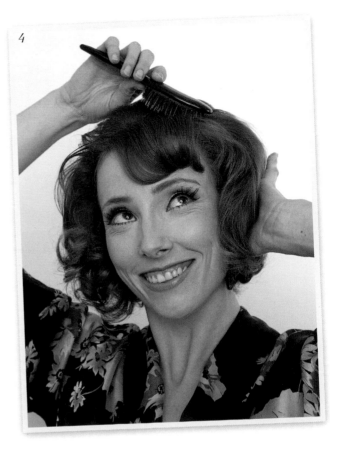

Step 5
Backcomb the sides and spray each section as before.

Step 6
Using a boar bristle brush, smooth the backcombing into shape (Fig. 4). Do this section by section, spraying each time you smooth the ends in place. Be careful not to comb out all of your backcombing. Use a pintail comb to lift areas that need to be heightened.

Step 7
Give everything a final spray with hairspray to hold.

This style looks lovely with a scarf tied as a hair band and knotted at the nape of your neck.

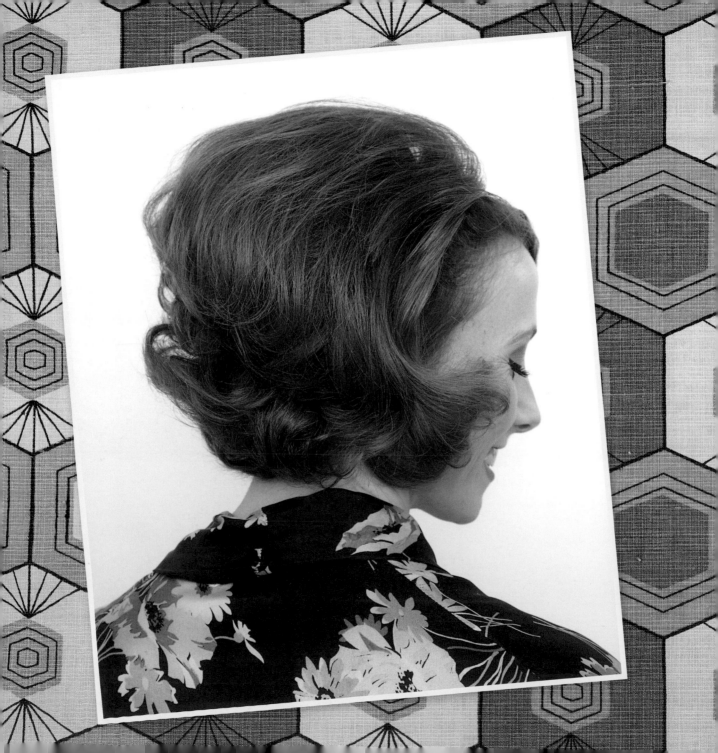

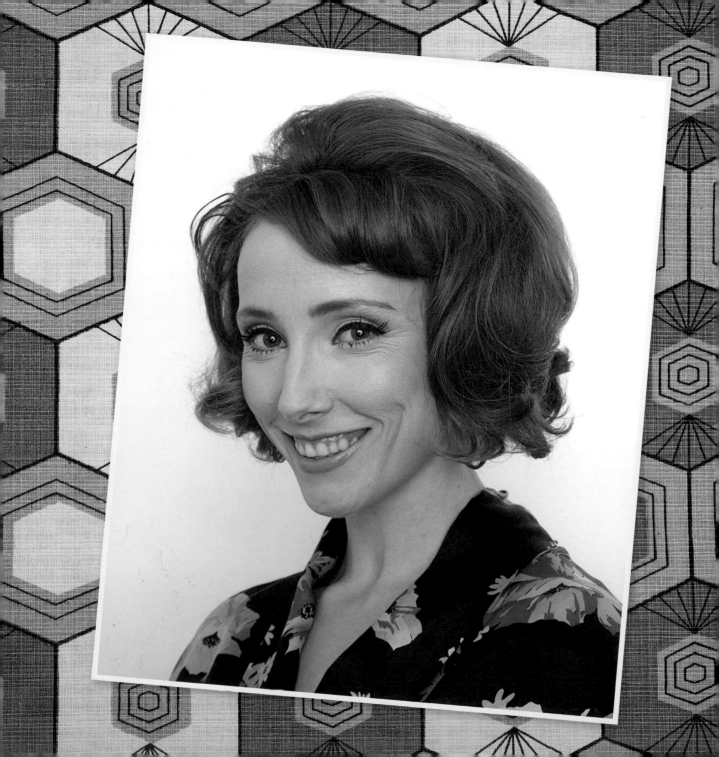

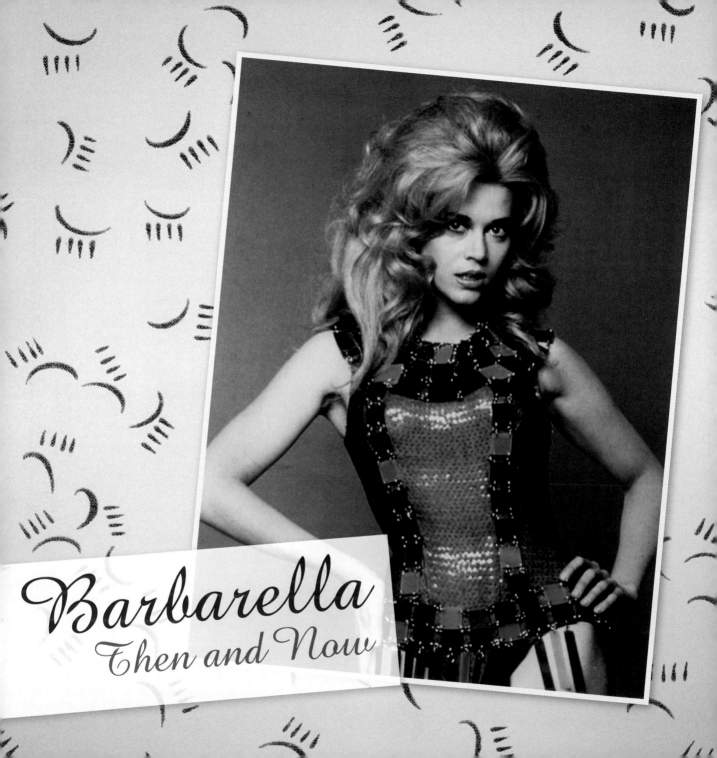

Barbarella
Then and Now

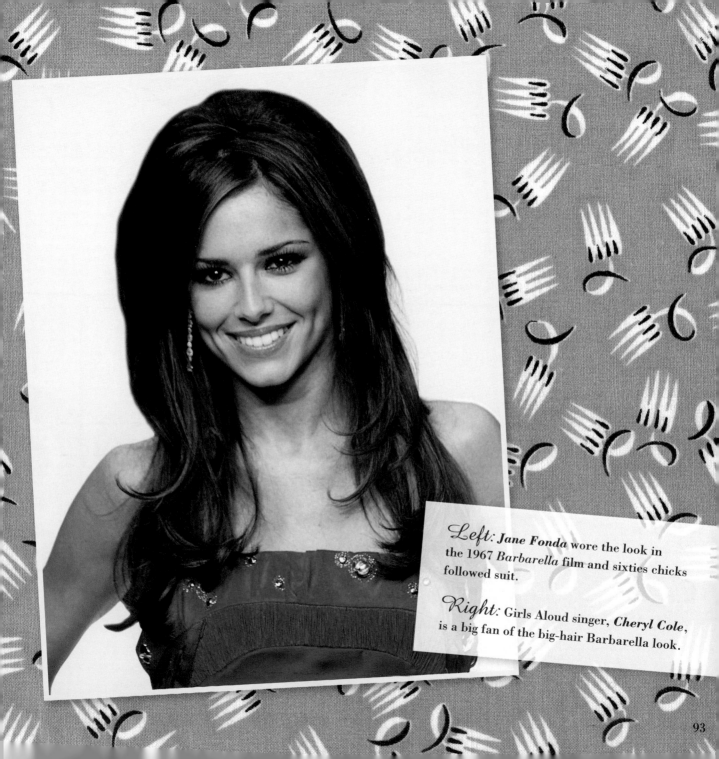

Left: **Jane Fonda** wore the look in the 1967 *Barbarella* film and sixties chicks followed suit.

Right: Girls Aloud singer, **Cheryl Cole**, is a big fan of the big-hair Barbarella look.

The Barbarella

The Barbarella is a giant wavy bouffant that is styled on long hair. A combination of the beehive and the shorter bouffant, it is often slightly tousled in style.

In the sixties, when big hair was the height of fashion, this style was featured in the adult *Barbarella* comic strip and was said to have been styled after Brigitte Bardot. Jane Fonda made the look iconic when she starred in the *Barbarella* film, which was released in 1968.

This hairstyle was a favourite of go-go dancers, with their knee high boots and miniskirts, who were first seen 'twisting' on the dance floors (and tables) of the United States in the early sixties.

You will need
Heated rollers or curling tongs
Comb
Boar bristle brush
Hair tie

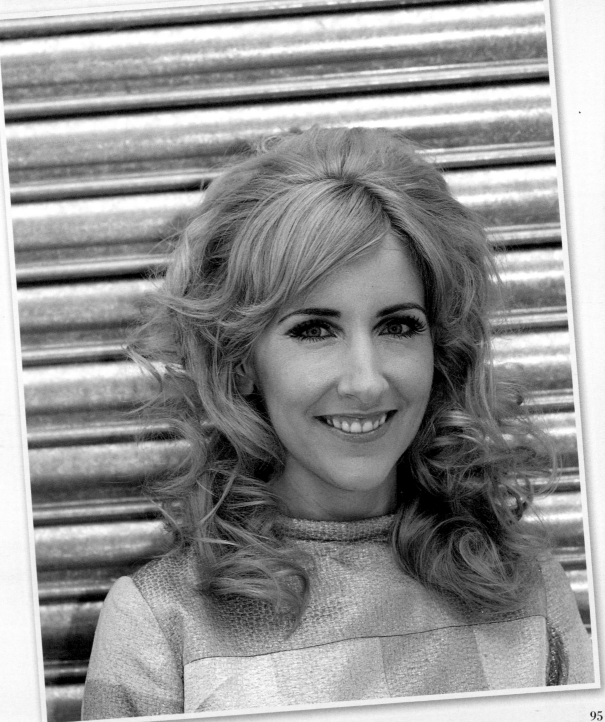

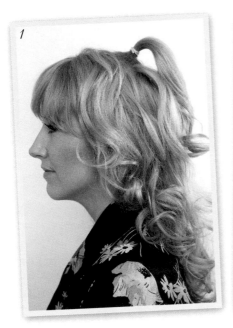

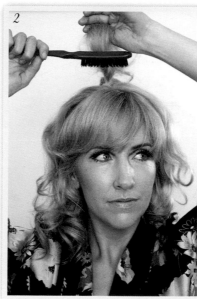

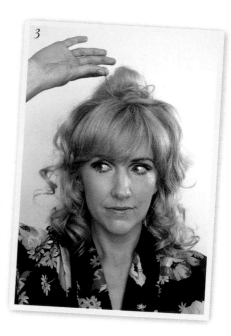

Step 1

Prep your hair using heated rollers and curling tongs to give as much volume as possible and also some curl. This is a big hairstyle – don't be afraid to make it as big as you can. It's easier to pat it down and make it smaller after backcombing.

Step 2

Take a diamond-shaped section of hair through your crown area and tie this into a ponytail (Fig. 1).

Step 3

Backcomb all of the hair in the ponytail (Fig. 2).

Step 4

Secure the backcombed ponytail with Kirby grips, arranging it in a bouffant-type shape (Fig. 3). This gives the style padding and height.

Step 5

Backcomb all the hair around the ponytail to give fullness. Then smooth the top section back with a boar bristle brush to cover your ponytail padding (Fig. 4).

Step 6

Backcomb your sides and some of the curls on the ends to create extra fullness. This will also help your finished style to hold. Give it all a generous burst of hairspray.

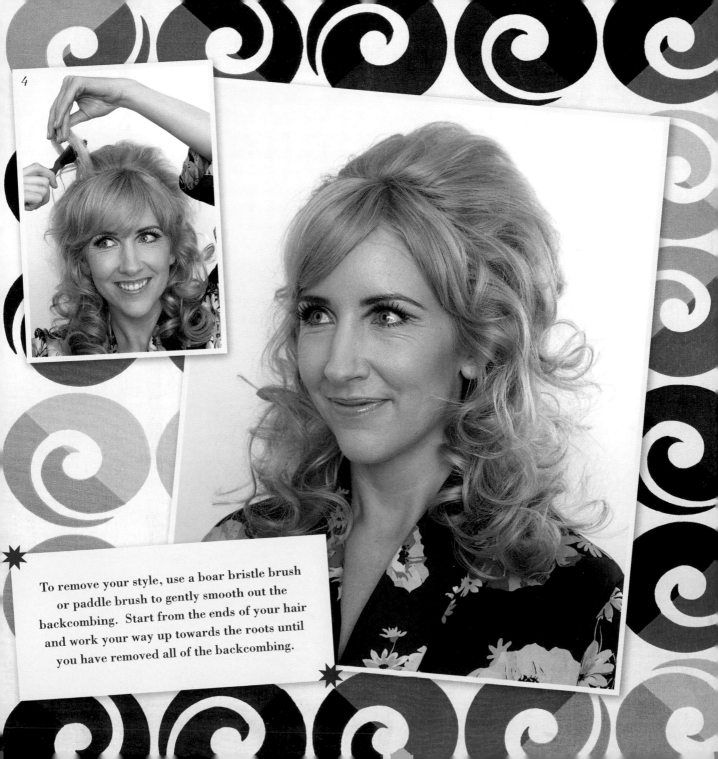

4

To remove your style, use a boar bristle brush or paddle brush to gently smooth out the backcombing. Start from the ends of your hair and work your way up towards the roots until you have removed all of the backcombing.

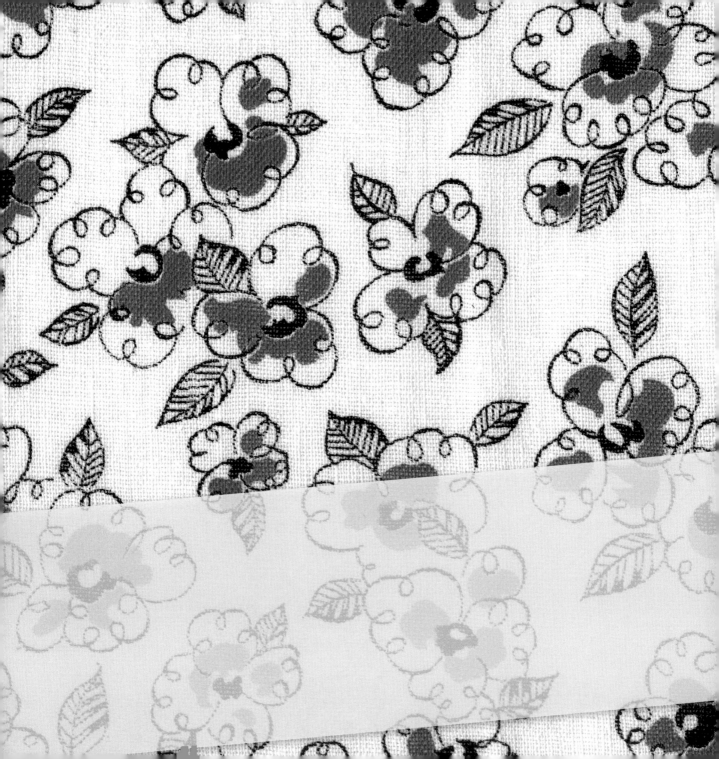

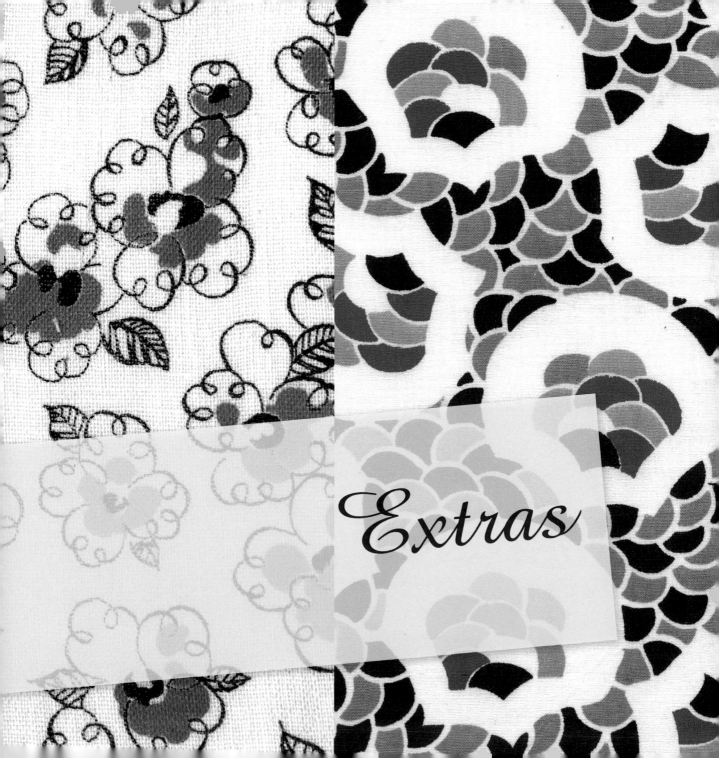

Extras

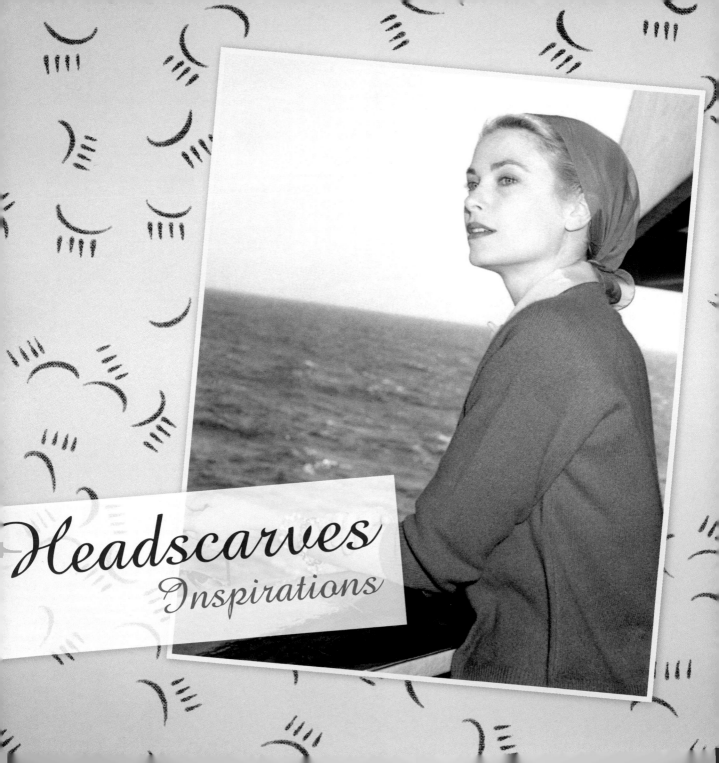

Headscarves
Inspirations

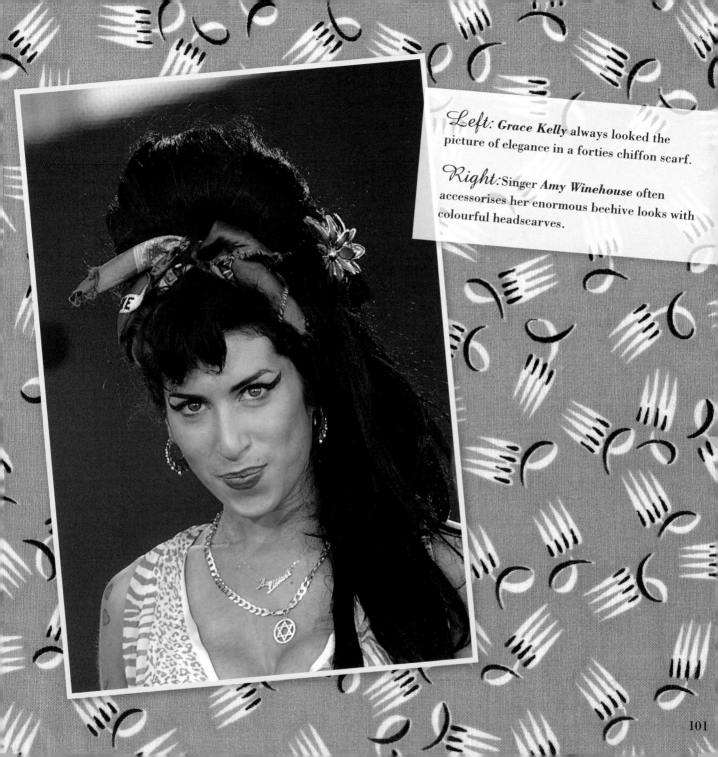

Left: *Grace Kelly* always looked the picture of elegance in a forties chiffon scarf.

Right: Singer *Amy Winehouse* often accessorises her enormous beehive looks with colourful headscarves.

Forties Headscarf

In the forties women would often spend all day with their hair in rollers. It didn't look especially nice to have rollers showing while going about daily business, so headscarves were the solution. These also protected hair from the elements. This particular way of tying a scarf was made famous by the war-time poster girl, Rosie the Riveter, Coronation Street's Hilda Ogden and, in recent years, has been seen on the likes of Amy Winehouse. It's a great way to hide your hair if you're having a bad hair day.

Step 1

Pin curl your hair or clip it up and out of the way.

Step 2

Take a triangular scarf (if you have a square scarf, simply fold it into a triangle). Place the long edge of the triangle at the nape of your neck and lay the scarf over the top of your head, with the short point of the triangle pointing towards your face. Take the other 2 points of the triangle and cross them over the top of your head and knot them into the start of a bow (Fig. 1).

Step 3

Take the short point of the triangle, place it over this first knot and continue tying the long points of the triangle into a bow (Fig. 2). Tuck the ends in if you like.

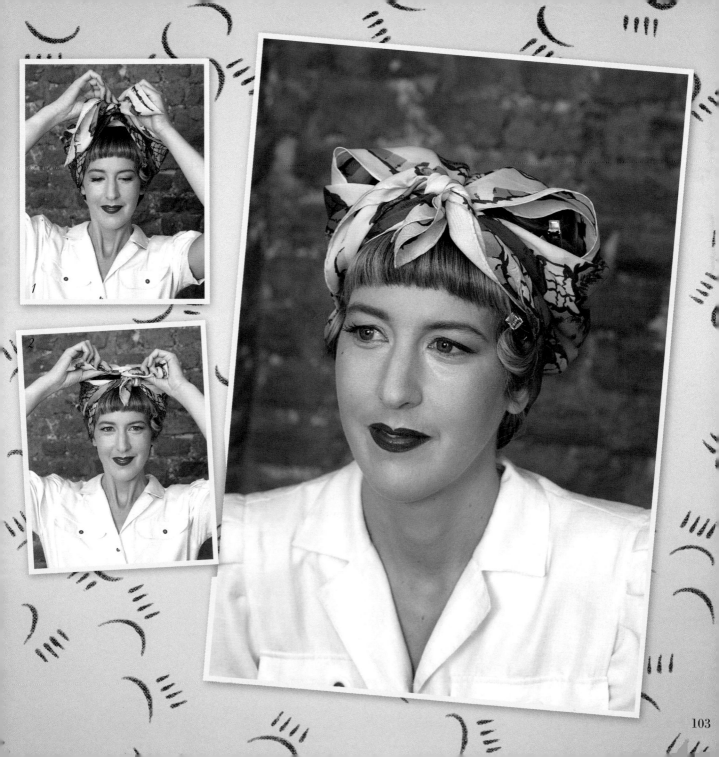

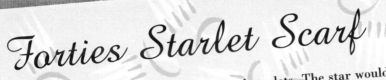

Forties Starlet Scarf

This style of scarf was frequently seen on Hollywood starlets. The star would tie her scarf as she sat in a Mustang convertible with the soft top down and her sunglasses on. The car would speed off, her beau driving, one hand on the steering wheel, one hand around her shoulder. Her perfect hair was thus protected from becoming an unsightly wind-blown mess and tangle.

This scarf was also made popular by the young Queen Elizabeth in the 1940s, as she was out riding her horses.

This one is very simple to do:

Take a triangular scarf (if it is square, fold it into a triangle). Place it over the top of your head with the shortest point facing the back. Tie the two longest points together under your chin.

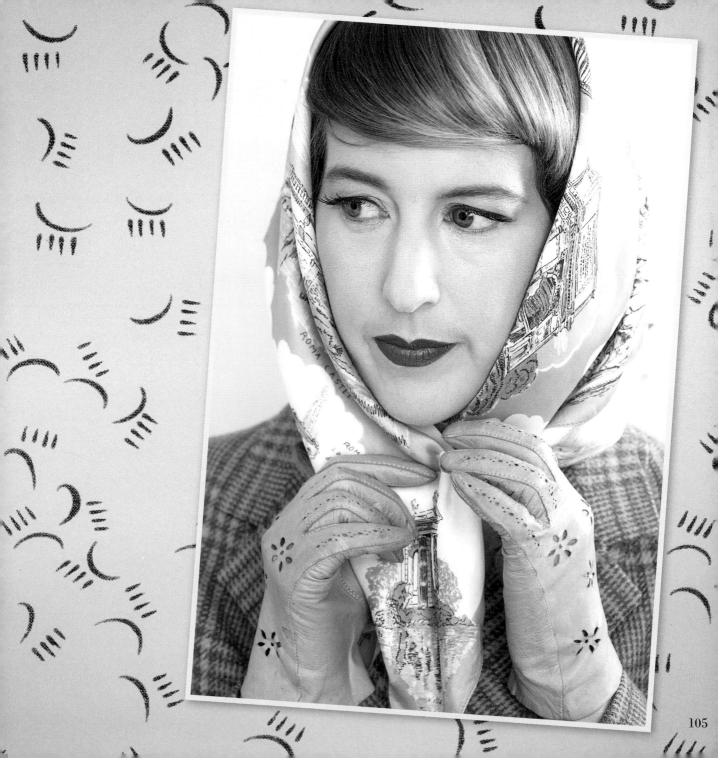

Fifties Ponytail Scarf

This scarf was a popular way for girls to brighten up their ponytail in the fifties. Tying a chiffon scarf around the base of your ponytail will also add an extra splash of colour to your outfit. Simply wrap a long, thin scarf around the ponytail and tie in a bow to secure. For an authentic fifties look, try also rolling your fringe under or quiff the front.

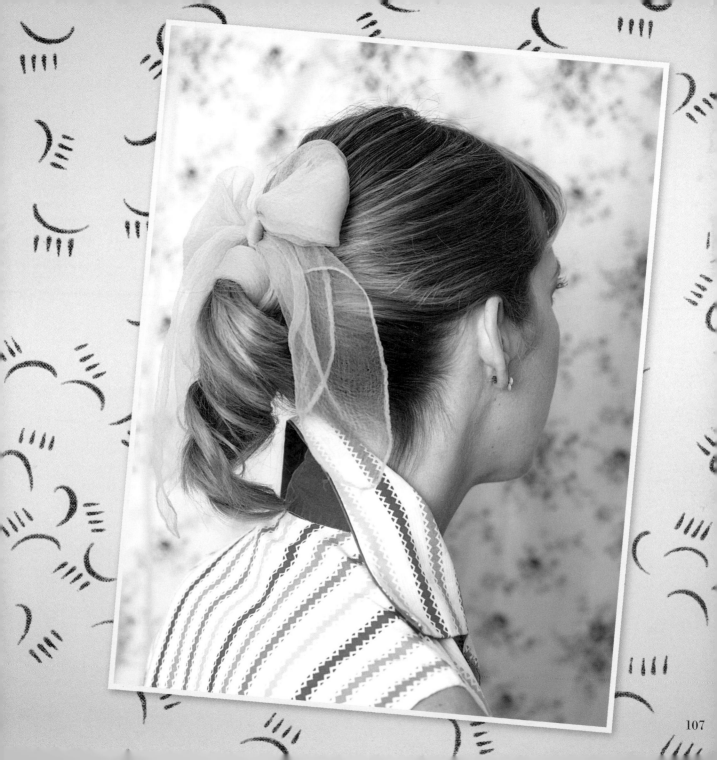

How to create padding

Hair padding, also known as a 'RAT', was historically made by women using thir own hair. They would collect this from their hair brushes and put it into a hairnet or an old stocking and then use the resulting pad to create extra volume, height and support for their gravity-defying styles. Padding is particularly useful for beehive hairstyles.

Nowadays you can easily make padding using hairwefts. Or you may find a ready-made pad, in the shape you want, made out of nylon or another synthetic product at a hairdressing suppliers.

To create your own padding, you need:

❋ **Hairwefts**
Either made from human hair or synthetic (synthetic is usually cheaper). You can find hairwefts at any hairdressing suppliers, on the internet, or perhaps your local chemist. Try to find a hairweft the same shade as your natural hair colour. That way, if you don't manage to cover your padding completely, your hairstyle will still look fabulous.

❋ **A hair net**
You can usually find these in the beauty section of your local chemist.

Step 1
Double over your hair net.

Step 2
Backcomb your hairweft to give it plenty of volume and place it inside your hair net.

Step 3
Adjust it to the shape you prefer (an oval shape usually works best) and use some thin cotton to sew the edges of the hair net together. There you have it!

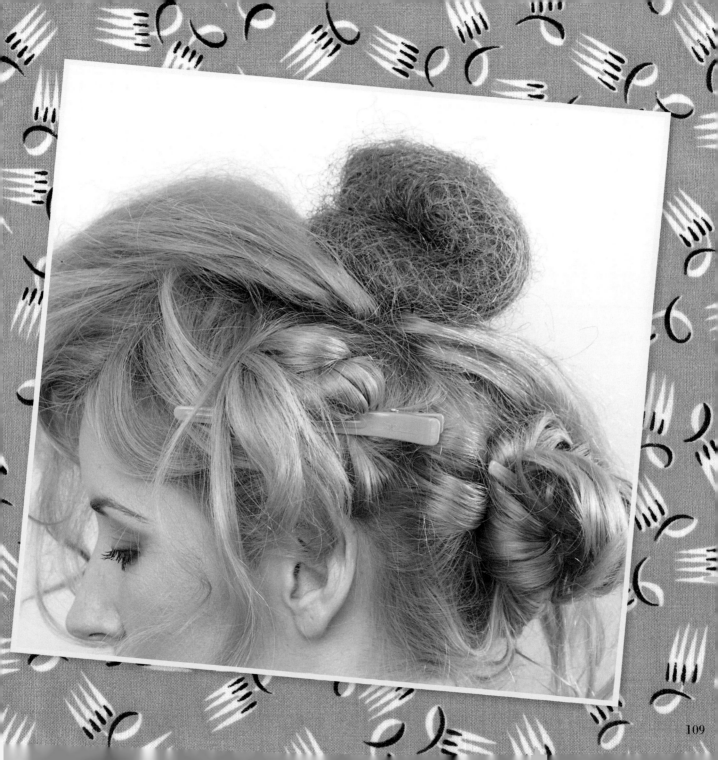

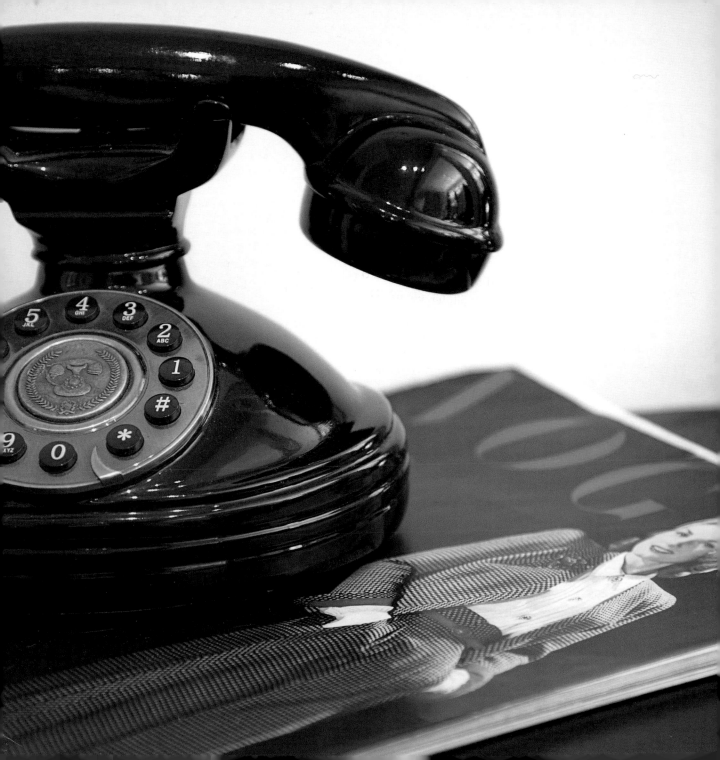

Picture Credits

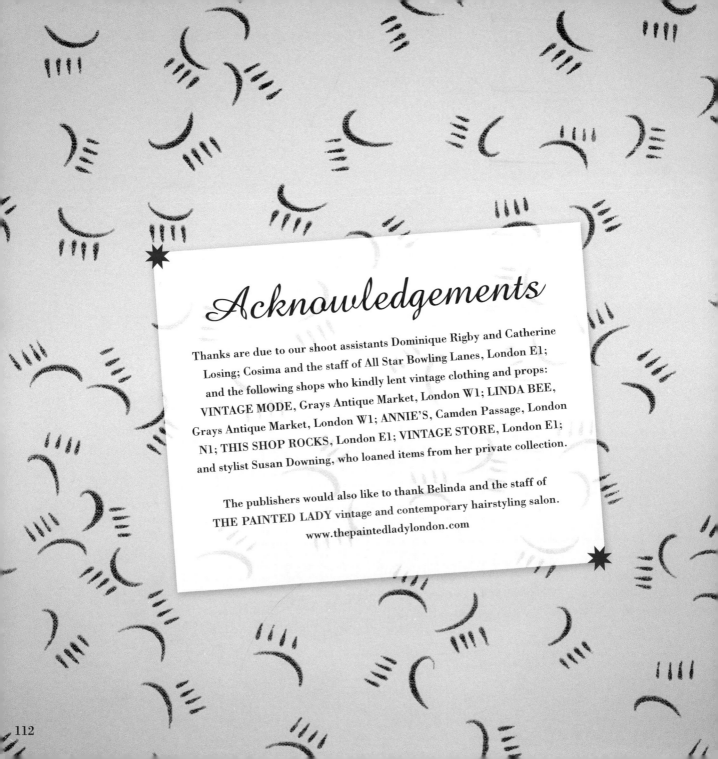

Acknowledgements

Thanks are due to our shoot assistants Dominique Rigby and Catherine Losing; Cosima and the staff of All Star Bowling Lanes, London E1; and the following shops who kindly lent vintage clothing and props: VINTAGE MODE, Grays Antique Market, London W1; LINDA BEE, Grays Antique Market, London W1; ANNIE'S, Camden Passage, London N1; THIS SHOP ROCKS, London E1; VINTAGE STORE, London E1; and stylist Susan Downing, who loaned items from her private collection.

The publishers would also like to thank Belinda and the staff of THE PAINTED LADY vintage and contemporary hairstyling salon. www.thepaintedladylondon.com